Overcoming Common Problems Series

Coping with Stammering
TRUDY STEWART AND JACKIE
TURNBULL

Coping with Stomach Ulcers
DR TOM SMITH

Coping with Strokes
DR TOM SMITH

Coping with Thrush
CAROLINE CLAYTON

Coping with Thyroid Problems
DR JOAN GOMEZ

Coping with Your Cervical Smear
KAREN EVENNETT

Crunch Points for Couples
JULIA COLE

Curing Arthritis – The Drug-Free Way
MARGARET HILLS

**Curing Arthritis – More ways to a
drug-free life**
MARGARET HILLS

Curing Arthritis Diet Book
MARGARET HILLS

Curing Arthritis Exercise Book
MARGARET HILLS AND JANET
HORWOOD

Cystic Fibrosis – A Family Affair
JANE CHUMBLEY

Depression
DR PAUL HAUCK

Depression at Work
VICKY MAUD

**Everything Parents Should Know
About Drugs**
SARAH LAWSON

Feverfew
DR STEWART JOHNSON

Gambling – A Family Affair
ANGELA WILLANS

Garlic
KAREN EVENNETT

Getting a Good Night's Sleep
FIONA JOHNSTON

The Good Stress Guide
MARY HARTLEY

Heart Attacks – Prevent and Survive
DR TOM SMITH

**Helping Children Cope with Attention
Deficit Disorder**
DR PATRICIA GILBERT

Helping Children Cope with Bullying
SARAH LAWSON

Helping Children Cope with Divorce
ROSEMARY WELLS

Helping Children Cope with Dyslexia
SALLY RAYMOND

Helping Children Cope with Grief
ROSEMARY WELLS

Helping Children Cope with Stammering
JACKIE TURNBULL AND TRUDY
STEWART

Hold Your Head Up High
DR PAUL HAUCK

How to Accept Yourself
DR WINDY DRYDEN

How to Be Your Own Best Friend
DR PAUL HAUCK

How to Cope when the Going Gets Tough
DR WINDY DRYDEN AND JACK
GORDON

How to Cope with Anaemia
DR JOAN GOMEZ

How to Cope with Bulimia
DR JOAN GOMEZ

How to Cope with Difficult Parents
DR WINDY DRYDEN AND JACK
GORDON

How to Cope with Difficult People
ALAN HOUEL WITH CHRISTIAN
GODEFROY

**How to Cope with People who Drive
You Crazy**
DR PAUL HAUCK

How to Cope with Splitting Up
VERA PEIFFER

How to Cope with Stress
DR PETER TYRER

How to Enjoy Your Retirement
VICKY MAUD

How to Improve Your Confidence
DR KENNETH HAMBLY

How to Interview and Be Interviewed
MICHELE BROWN AND GYLES
BRANDRETH

How to Keep Your Cholesterol in Check
DR ROBERT POVEY

How to Love and Be Loved
DR PAUL HAUCK

How to Pass Your Driving Test
DONALD RIDLAND

How to Raise Confident Children
CAROLE BALDOCK

How to Stand up for Yourself
DR PAUL HAUCK

Overcoming Common Problems Series

How to Start a Conversation and Make Friends
DON GABOR

How to Stick to a Diet
DEBORAH STEINBERG AND
DR WINDY DRYDEN

How to Stop Worrying
DR FRANK TALLIS

How to Succeed as a Single Parent
CAROLE BALDOCK

How to Untangle Your Emotional Knots
DR WINDY DRYDEN AND JACK
GORDON

How to Write a Successful CV
JOANNA GUTMANN

Hysterectomy
SUZIE HAYMAN

The Irritable Bowel Diet Book
ROSEMARY NICOL

The Irritable Bowel Stress Book
ROSEMARY NICOL

Is HRT Right for You?
DR ANNE MACGREGOR

Jealousy
DR PAUL HAUCK

Learning to Live with Multiple Sclerosis
DR ROBERT POVEY, ROBIN DOWIE
AND GILLIAN PRETT

Living with Angina
DR TOM SMITH

Living with Asthma
DR ROBERT YOUNGSON

Living with Crohn's Disease
DR JOAN GOMEZ

Living with Diabetes
DR JOAN GOMEZ

Living with Grief
DR TONY LAKE

Living with High Blood Pressure
DR TOM SMITH

Living with Nut Allergies
KAREN EVENNETT

Living with Osteoporosis
DR JOAN GOMEZ

Living with a Stoma
DR CRAIG WHITE

Menopause
RAEWYN MACKENZIE

The Migraine Diet Book
SUE DYSON

Motor Neurone Disease – A Family Affair
DR DAVID OLIVER

Overcoming Anger
DR WINDY DRYDEN

Overcoming Anxiety
DR WINDY DRYDEN

Overcoming Guilt
DR WINDY DRYDEN

Overcoming Jealousy
DR WINDY DRYDEN

Overcoming Procrastination
DR WINDY DRYDEN

Overcoming Shame
DR WINDY DRYDEN

Overcoming Your Addictions
DR WINDY DRYDEN AND
DR WALTER MATWEYCHUK

The Parkinson's Disease Handbook
DR RICHARD GODWIN-AUSTEN

The PMS Diet Book
KAREN EVENNETT

A Positive Thought for Every Day
DR WINDY DRYDEN

Second Time Around
ANNE LOVELL

Serious Mental Illness – A Family Affair
GWEN HOWE

Sex and Relationships
ROSEMARY STONES

The Stress Workbook
JOANNA GUTMANN

The Subfertility Handbook
VIRGINIA IRONSIDE AND SARAH
BIGGS

Talking About Anorexia
How to cope with life without starving
MAROUSHKA MONRO

Talking with Confidence
DON GABOR

Ten Steps to Positive Living
DR WINDY DRYDEN

Think Your Way to Happiness
DR WINDY DRYDEN AND JACK
GORDON

The Travellers' Good Health Guide
TED LANKESTER

Understanding Obsessions and Compulsions
A self-help manual
DR FRANK TALLIS

Understanding Your Personality
Myers-Briggs and more
PATRICIA HEDGES

Overcoming Common Problems

Living with Nut Allergies

Karen Evennett

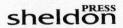

Published in Great Britain in 2000 by
Sheldon Press
Holy Trinity Church
Marylebone Road
London NW1 4DU

British Library Cataloguing-in-Publication Data

A catalogue record for this book is available from the British Library

ISBN 0–85969–835–1

Typeset by Deltatype Limited, Birkenhead, Merseyside
Printed in Great Britain by
Biddles Ltd, Guildford and King's Lynn

Contents

Part One

1 Friend or Foe?   3
2 Allergy and the Immune System   7
3 The Symptoms of Anaphylaxis   13
4 Living With Your Allergy   19
5 Troubleshooting   30
6 Other Allergic Conditions   37
7 Nut-free Nutrition   46

Part Two: Recipes

Starters   56
Salads   61
Main Dishes   66
Pasta and Rice   72
Side Dishes   78

Useful Addresses   81
Further Reading   82
Index   83

Acknowledgement

The author would like to acknowledge the help provided by the Anaphylaxis Campaign in supplying information about allergies in general and nut allergy in particular. The Campaign provides ongoing help and information for people with severe food allergies. Contact Anaphylaxis Campaign, PO Box 149, Fleet, Hampshire GU13 0FA. Tel. 01252 542029. Website: www.anaphylaxis.org.uk

PART ONE

1

Friend or Foe?

Think back to the 1970s when vegetarianism was taking off. No meat-free cook book was complete without a decent helping of nutty recipes. Nut roasts, stuffings and cutlets were a brilliant alternative to meat, providing vitamins B6 and E, calcium, phosphorus, magnesium, niacin (vitamin B3), iron, zinc, copper, selenium and essential fatty acids.

There's no doubt about it – nuts are extremely good for you. In a culture where 80 per cent of children aged two to 11 get less than their daily requirement of three major nutrients – calcium, iron and zinc – a sprinkling of nuts in their salad, or a dollop of peanut butter on their bread are seen as health promoting.

Adults benefit from eating nuts, too. Just 100 g daily of peanuts will give you all the niacin (vitamin B3) you need to improve your levels of the healthy (HDL or High Density Lipoprotein) type of cholesterol that protects your heart from disease.

But here's the irony. The vogue for eating nuts has highlighted the fact that they can trigger a fatal allergic reaction.

In October 1993, 17-year-old Sarah Reading died after eating a lemon meringue pie served to her in the restaurant of a well-known department store. Sarah suffered anaphylaxis – an extreme allergic reaction in which the blood pressure falls dramatically and the patient rapidly loses consciousness. The dessert contained peanut – to which Sarah was fatally allergic. Her tragic death exposed the fact that just a small amount of peanut could kill someone like her – and, furthermore, that peanuts could turn up where you wouldn't expect to find them.

It soon became clear to Sarah's family that the condition from which she died was by no means rare. Consequently the Anaphylaxis Campaign was launched in January 1994 by a small group of parents, including Sarah's father David. Immediately the newly formed Campaign became inundated with calls for advice and information. The vast majority of these enquiries came from the parents of children who suffer serious allergic reactions to peanuts, tree nuts, or both. Occasionally other foods and substances were implicated, such as milk, eggs, soya, sesame, shellfish, insect stings and natural rubber (latex). In many cases there had been life-threatening episodes, yet often the people concerned had received minimal medical advice. It became crystal clear to the Campaign that information is the key to managing severe allergies. If Sarah Reading had been well informed, and had been carrying medication to treat a severe allergic reaction, she would probably be alive today.

Tragically, the deaths continue – still due to lack of information. In 1998, Laura Thrasher, a 19-year-old student, died after suffering an overwhelming allergic reaction to nuts in a dessert during her first night at Cambridge University. And, in 1999, the 21-year-old athlete Ross Baillie suffered a devastating allergic reaction when he bit into a coronation chicken sandwich after working out with swimming champion Mark Foster at Bath University. Ross was taken to a university health centre where adrenaline was administered, but too much time had elapsed, and he slipped into a coma and died three days later in the Royal United Hospital at Bath.

By the time of Ross Baillie's tragic premature death, the Anaphylaxis Campaign had attracted 5,400 members, but prominent allergists are confident that this is just the tip of the iceberg.

Peanuts are the most common cause of life-threatening anaphylaxis in the UK, but tree nuts (such as walnuts, brazils, almonds, hazels or cashews) can also be responsible, as can seeds – and particularly sesame seeds, which are becoming a growing problem as they become a bigger part of our health-conscious twenty-first-century diet. Not everyone with a peanut allergy will also be allergic to sesame seeds, or vice versa. However, the allergies do overlap in some people. Chestnuts, curiously, tend to overlap with latex allergy (another common cause of anaphylaxis) in some people. The Anaphylaxis Campaign says we may see a growth in severe reactions to other seed products (sunflower seeds, and spices such as fennel, cumin, and caraway seeds) as they become a bigger part of our diet. Poppy seeds are already becoming a more common problem for the British as they have started to appear quite routinely on continental breads and pastries. However, it is impossible to predict whether these allergies will ever be as widespread as peanut allergy, which has only been a big problem since peanuts have become such a commonplace ingredient in everything from Indian, Thai and Chinese dishes to breads, cakes and desserts.

Strictly speaking the peanut is not actually a nut, but a legume. The average American eats roughly 5 kg (11 lb) of peanut products every year. About half of this is made up of peanut butter, while the remainder comes from cakes, cookies, puddings and sweets. The rest of us may not be quite so peanut-hungry, but, all over the world, peanuts are extremely popular. And the increase in peanut-induced anaphylaxis may be partly due to the early age at which children are being given them. A piece of bread with a scraping of peanut butter may seem like a lovely first finger food to offer a baby, but by giving peanuts to very young children, we may be setting up the mechanism that could one day lead to life-threatening anaphylaxis.

A recent study at the Isle of Wight Allergy Research Unit found that one in 75 children had been sensitized to peanuts by the age of four. In some, the allergy may remain latent, but at least half will experience symptoms. Extrapolated across the UK, this suggests that many thousands of children are affected.

The risk of sensitization to a food is higher if you come from a family that is atopic – that is to say, has a tendency to develop allergies such as hay fever, eczema and asthma. Having an atopic tendency doesn't mean you will definitely be allergic to nuts, but you are more susceptible.

We know basically what happens when someone becomes allergic to something. When they first encounter the food or substance, they may have no visible reaction to it. However, their immune system makes a note that this is an enemy – and it prepares their body to deal with it by reacting (often violently as in anaphylaxis) whenever it is re-encountered.

In many cases, children appear to have reacted to peanuts at the first known exposure. This has raised the possibility – supported by research – that these youngsters may have been sensitized to peanut proteins present in the mother's breast milk after she had eaten peanuts. Alternatively, these children may have been sensitized in the womb where peanut proteins ingested by the mother crossed the placenta.

If this is true, mothers may be able to minimize the chances of their children developing food allergies by manipulating their diet in pregnancy and while breastfeeding. However, further research is needed so that the mechanisms of sensitization can be better understood. Any dietary manipulation would have to be done in consultation with a registered dietitian.

In this book I aim to convey the message that food-induced anaphylaxis is serious, but it is most certainly manageable. Where those affected have proper guidance, are prescribed appropriate treatments, and commit themselves to being vigilant whenever food is around, they are highly unlikely to suffer a fatal reaction. I intend to answer the common questions asked in relation to food allergy, particularly nut allergy. How do I cope if I'm affected? And how can life be made easier for those of us with nut allergies? Later on in the book is a chapter on nut-free nutrition, aimed particularly at vegetarians, and a selection of recipes which I hope will fire your imagination and encourage you to broaden your diet to get all the goodness you would otherwise get from nuts without having to go anywhere near them.

2

Allergy and the Immune System

Your immune system is a sophisticated network of glands and hormones that defends the body against foreign organisms (such as bacteria, viruses and parasites) and guards against the growth of cancers. When your body comes under attack by germs, your immune system is designed to put you out of action with fever and achiness so that more energy can go towards fighting the infection. It's your own body that's making you feel so grotty – not the invading virus – but if your immune system can do its job quickly, this is a sign that it's strong and healthy. For the short time you're laid up, your immune system is stopping the invading cells from reproducing, and removing any toxins left in its wake. A slower recovery means the invaders are continuing to get past your immune system, so it's not working as well as it should.

Your lymph nodes act as a meeting point for white cells when infection strikes. From the nodes they'll be despatched to protect any affected tissues needing help. If you think you're over an infection, because you can no longer feel the symptoms, but your lymph nodes are still swollen, this is a sign that you have an infection your immune system isn't managing to shift.

Similarly, when you cut yourself, the area is likely to become swollen – a sign that immune cells and antibodies are flooding to the area's defence. Any pus that oozes from the scene is made up of dead white cells, germs and other debris which are left behind after you've fought off any infection to the wound. A slow-healing wound that weeps on and off for several weeks is a sign that your white cells aren't able to fight the infection off.

Like any part of the body, the immune system can go wrong – and a defective immune system provides fewer defences against infection than it should. But a hypersensitive immune system overreacts to certain substances that should not normally be seen as invaders, because they should carry no threat to your health. This is allergy. But, although woeful if you suffer with it, a hypersensitive immune system need not be as hazardous as a defective one.

What happens when you're allergic?

Nuts are good for most people – we have seen all the good they can do in the last chapter. But, if your body has decided the nut is Enemy Number One, an alarm bell will ring at any sniff of contact with one, and, just as antibodies normally sweep into action to fight bacteria and viruses, a special group of antibodies now comes into play.

Found in blood serum, immunoglobulins (the scientific word for antibodies) are divided into five groups.

Immunoglobulin E (IgE) is the allergy antibody. People who do not have allergies normally have only small amounts of IgE, but can produce more as a response to parasites such as worms. People with allergies readily produce large amounts of IgE.

The other groups are:

- IgG, the most abundant antibody, forming 75 per cent of the total serum immunoglobulin level, is active in response to bacteria and viruses. It's the memory antibody, forming usually lifelong memories of attackers. It is also recognized as the 'blocking antibody' capable of preventing IgE from triggering allergic response.
- IgA, found in tears, sweat and saliva, defends us against micro-organisms which might invade our digestive and respiratory systems.
- IgM is a temporary antibody formed when a new attacker invades your body. It gives way to IgG for longer-term response.
- IgD is a mystery antibody – we know it's there, but we do not know what it does.

Types of allergic reaction

- Type 1 is the immediate response normally associated with allergy. It involves IgE which triggers the release of powerful chemicals from body cells causing anaphylaxis, asthma, hay fever, eczema and urticaria (nettle rash).
- Type 2 includes autoimmune disorders (where the immune system starts to attack the body's own tissues).
- Type 3 includes adverse reactions in tissues.
- Type 4 is a delayed sensitivity to an allergen.

In both immune and allergic responses, the white cells are the big

8

players. These are divided into T cells (which originate in the thymus gland), and B cells (which mature in the bone marrow). They circulate through the blood and tissue, functioning for as long as 20 years, and developing a remarkable memory for things they should attack, while producing many millions of different antibodies, each specific to individual invading substances (antigens).

When the immune system is acting in defence, the T cells attack the antigens and activate other cells to defend the body, while the B cells produce antibodies in the blood. When a hypersensitive immune system reacts, a small number of B cells are ready to react to the substance before they've even encountered it. When the substance comes their way for the first time, it 'locks into' the specific B cells for which it has an affinity. This causes the B cells to divide, some of the progeny becoming plasma cells which secrete and then produce antibodies. The level of IgE in the blood serum rises but drops after a few weeks as plasma cells can only live for a short time. The process constitutes sensitization, however, and, although it does not give rise to symptoms because the number of cells involved is so small, some of the B cells will survive as long-living memory cells, which are primed to react far more violently on their next encounter with the same allergen.

The degree of severity of subsequent reactions will vary between individual people, and your own reaction to an allergen will not be identical on every occasion. There are many factors which alter its severity – and your allergy may grow weaker (or stronger) with time. But once you have developed an allergy, your immune system maintains a memory of the responsible allergen in the form of antibodies, and you cannot trick it into forgetting about the allergen by avoiding nuts (if these are what affect you) for a year or so. The main exception to this is when an allergy develops early in childhood. As the immune system is then rather immature, its memory is not quite as good. Therefore most children outgrow their food allergies. Even nut allergy is outgrown in a small number of cases.

Allergy tests

All people suspected of being at risk of anaphylaxis should be referred to an allergy clinic. But once a referral is made, the patient is plagued by questions. Is skin-prick testing dangerous? At what age can testing be given? Are the tests that are offered reliable? In this section, we attempt to answer these and other common questions.

Diagnosis of allergy depends on a combination of three factors:

1 A detailed history of past allergic reactions and other allergic conditions, such as asthma, eczema and hay fever, and consideration of any seasonal or environmental symptoms.
2 A thorough medical examination, involving peak flow measurements if the patient is asthmatic, and a close look to see if there are allergic symptoms in the skin, eyes and nose. This information will help the specialist decide which tests are appropriate.
3 Results of allergy tests – usually skin-prick testing or blood testing.

Skin-prick tests

These are suitable for any age group; even babies under a year old are tested at some clinics in this way. A tiny prick is made with a lancet through a drop of allergen placed on the skin, usually on the forearm.

A positive reaction will be indicated by itching within a few minutes. The site where the allergen was introduced then becomes red and swollen, with a raised weal in the centre that looks like a nettle sting. The weal enlarges and reaches its maximum size within 15–20 minutes, when the measurements of the weal are recorded. The reaction fades within an hour.

A negative response usually means the patient is not sensitive to that allergen. But skin-prick testing for food allergens may be unreliable and 'false negatives' can occur where the reaction to food is not immediate. A negative response may occur if the patient is taking antihistamines and these should be stopped three to five days before testing (it is important to talk with your doctor about this).

A positive response usually means the patient is allergic to that allergen. However, a patient may have a positive skin test but suffer no symptoms when coming into contact with the allergen. Positive skin tests may occur before symptoms have become apparent. Skin tests may also remain positive to foods and inhalants even when the patient has grown out of allergic symptoms.

Blood tests

RAST (Radioallergosorbent test) and CAP-RAST are the most commonly used blood tests in the UK (the CAP-RAST seems to be superseding the RAST test because it appears to be more reliable and more sensitive). Other immunological blood tests using not radioactive material but enzymes are now superseding the original RAST methodology. Blood tests give graded results from 1 to 6, with 6 being the most positive. Blood tests are not affected by antihistamines, and can be used in patients with severe eczema. However they are quite costly and the results are not available immediately.

Looking after your immune system

The fact that you have a hypersensitive immune system is no excuse not to look after it. Recovery from any illness is more rapid if your immune system is in good condition, and this may include your recovery from allergic reactions.

To this end:

- Exercise regularly – 30 to 45 minutes of moderately intense aerobic exercise (walking, cycling or dancing) three times a week is all it takes to enhance your resistance to upper respiratory tract infections.
- Cut down on stress – it's one of the greatest threats to the immune system. Exercise – especially outdoors – is a good stress reliever. Yoga and meditation will also help you relax and put stress in perspective.
- Eat yogurt. People who regularly eat live yogurt appear to have stronger immune systems. US research has found that eating it increases our production of gamma-interferon, a protein that boosts the immune response.
- Use less sugar. Eating a lot of sugar reduces the ability of your white cells to engulf and destroy bacteria. Alcohol has also been shown to increase susceptibility to infections.
- Get a good night's sleep to boost your immune system. In one study, 42 healthy volunteers were allowed only four hours of sleep – afterwards they had suffered a 30 per cent drop in the natural killer cells which fight infection.
- Eat a well-balanced diet. Include at least two to four servings of fruit and three to five servings of vegetables every day to provide your body with optimal amounts of nutrients and keep your immune system strong.
- Don't be afraid to show emotion. Crying easily is a healthy sign. The stress hormone cortisol is shed in tears – so take the opportunity of having a good sob when you feel comfortable

doing so. If you find it difficult to cry, try watching a weepy movie to get you going. Bottled-up sadness will be released along with your tears for the film.

Another healthy emotion is laughter, which raises levels of immunoglobulin A, an antibody in the mucous lining of the nasal cavity, and helps release hormonal substances called cytokines that promote the activity of 'natural killer' white blood cells which fight off invading bacteria and viruses.

3
The Symptoms of Anaphylaxis

Up to a million people across the UK experience severe allergic reactions to foods or other substances, such as insect venom or drugs. As stated previously, the condition is known as anaphylaxis. Peanuts and tree nuts are the foods most commonly implicated in the UK and for that reason they have tended to capture the headlines. Although some of the reporting has been inaccurate and sensationalist, there is no doubt that nut allergy should be taken very seriously. Would you know what to do in the event of a severe allergic reaction?

First of all, it is vital that if you consider that you, or your child, may be at risk of anaphylaxis, you should see your GP and seek a referral to an NHS allergy clinic. With proper guidance, you can learn to recognize the symptoms of anaphylaxis and will be able to treat them should they occur.

The symptoms of anaphylaxis may include some or all of the following:

- tingling of the lips or in the mouth;
- swelling of the lips, throat or mouth;
- difficulty in swallowing or speaking;
- flushing of the skin or generalized rash;
- abdominal cramps, nausea, vomiting and diarrhoea;
- wheezy chest;
- feeling of faintness and impending doom.

Symptoms may appear within seconds or minutes of exposure, but can take over an hour. The early features of an acute allergic reaction do not always progress to anaphylaxis, but you should remain alert to this possibility – particularly if nuts are the trigger. The symptoms may worsen rapidly.

- The lining of your upper airways (the larynx and trachea) may become increasingly swollen, narrowing the space through which oxygen can pass.
- Breathing in may produce a harsh rasping sound called stridor. When the lining of the lower airways (the bronchi and bron-

chioles) becomes swollen, breathing out produces a wheeze, like a feeble bagpipe.

- Blood vessels in your circulatory system may become leaky, reducing the volume of blood in your arteries, veins and heart, leading to a fast but faint pulse. This reduced blood supply will make you feel faint, and, ultimately, leads to unconsciousness, shock and on rare occasions death.

Even if symptoms triggered by nuts have always been mild – such as a tingling in the mouth – it's vital you recognize that this is likely to be an allergy and you should ask your GP to refer you to an allergy specialist so that any risk – should it exist – can be evaluated.

If you are considered to be at risk of a severe reaction, you need to know how to treat the symptoms. The front-line treatment is injected adrenaline, also known as epinephrine. The name adrenaline will be used throughout this book, but it is important to remember that there is a likelihood of the alternative name replacing it throughout the world.

Adrenaline is a hormone that your body produces naturally from your adrenal glands (situated just above your kidneys). It's the hormone that controls your fight or flight response – helping you get away from danger – and it's pumped into your bloodstream in response to fear. In a dangerous situation, you become pale as the blood which would colour your skin is redirected to your muscles to give you the choice of staying and fighting, or running away. Your heart starts beating faster to make sure your muscles get an adequate supply of blood.

During an allergic reaction, your adrenal glands snap into action, pumping out adrenaline to help you fight the allergic process by constricting your blood vessels and preventing them from becoming leaky. However, in a severe attack, the reaction can overwhelm the counteracting effects of adrenaline, and the only way to outweigh the effects of the anaphylaxis is to introduce more adrenaline into the body.

Adrenaline can be administered by injection, or by inhalation, but is not taken orally as medicine. The best way of taking it is by injection. Inhaled adrenaline can be effective for mild or moderate symptoms involving the mouth, throat or respiratory system, but there is no adrenaline inhaler licensed for use in the UK (although some doctors prescribe an imported device on a 'named patient basis').

When a reaction starts, stay very alert. As we have seen, anaphylaxis can develop with little warning and it is essential to act sooner rather than later if you suspect you may be having a severe reaction. If you know you are at risk from a life-threatening reaction, you should be carrying at least two pre-loaded adrenaline injections on you at all times. These are prescribed by your doctor and are extremely effective in treating the symptoms of severe allergy. When to inject is a matter of judgement and hopefully you will be able to discuss this in advance with your GP or consultant.

Key questions are: Is there a marked difficulty in breathing or swallowing? Is there sudden weakness or floppiness? Is there a steady deterioration? Any of these are signs of a serious reaction and most experts would agree that adrenaline should be administered without delay.

With the injector positioned correctly, an injection will deliver a full dose straight into the muscle in the side of the thigh. In the vast majority of cases, adrenaline will work effectively to halt or relieve your symptoms and buy you time until medical help arrives.

If you do not have adrenaline with you, get emergency medical help in the fastest way possible.

Check your adrenaline supplies regularly. Adrenaline which is more than about three months past its expiry date may be ineffective. The colour of your adrenaline should be clear, like water. If it has yellow or brown discolouration or particles floating in it, it shouldn't be used.

Emergency action

1 If you suspect you're having a bad reaction – or what may be the start of a bad reaction – use your adrenaline kit.
2 Someone must call 999 and give the following information: 'It is an emergency. The patient is suffering from suspected anaphylaxis.'
3 The caller should give the address the ambulance is being called to, with the postcode if known.
4 Someone should wait outside the building to direct the ambulance crew to the patient.
5 When the ambulance crew arrives, repeat that the patient is suffering from suspected anaphylaxis. Tell them what has been administered.

6 If there is no improvement in symptoms after five minutes, and the ambulance hasn't arrived, a second adrenaline shot can be administered. This is why it is important to carry two injection kits if you are known or suspected to be at risk of severe reactions.

Trish's story

Peanut allergy can be very serious. But I didn't know this when my health visitor suggested I built up my son, Sam, with peanut butter sandwiches. He was one year old, weighed just 12 lbs, and looked like a walking skeleton. My husband Kevin, 36, and I had tried everything to get him to put on weight. But he seemed to be allergic to most baby foods, and by his first birthday he was living on a diet of carrots and breast milk. Despite his allergies to other foods, we had a hard job persuading our doctor that Sam was allergic. But when Kevin heard that the health visitor had suggested feeding Sam peanut butter, alarm bells rang. 'Don't risk it, love!' he said. 'I read somewhere that people with allergies should avoid peanuts like the plague.' That was the first time I was alerted to the possible problems with peanuts.

About six months later, our older children – Lynsey, eight, and Ryan, six – were eating peanuts and they left the bag open where Sam could get it.

Suddenly there was mayhem as Lynsey came running into the kitchen shouting, 'Sam's got a nut in his mouth!' I'd seen a *That's Life* programme about kids choking on nuts, and charged into the sitting room to fish it out. I retrieved it in one piece, but, within seconds, Sam started to make a weird wheezing noise and his entire body erupted in white lumps.

These went down without me having to call the doctor, and I put it down to yet another allergy. But a few months later we were on holiday on the Isle of Wight when Sam picked up and licked a peanut from a tray. I didn't see him do it – I just heard that awful noise again, and rushed him to the loo, where, already, his arms were completely covered in white lumps.

Back home, I decided we had to see the doctor about this. He agreed to give Sam a blood test, and this came back with a positive result for peanut allergy.

Within a week I'd contacted an allergy support group and got

Sam an appointment with a specialist in Leicester. My blood ran cold as I heard the low-down on peanut allergy – that reactions can be unpredictable and even life-threatening.

But we were relieved to learn that severe allergic reactions are treatable. We were given emergency medication to treat any future reactions: antihistamine for mild reactions and injectable adrenaline in case Sam ever has a life-threatening reaction. So far, we've been lucky – that hasn't happened. But I have to watch Sam like a hawk. He doesn't go to parties without me. And, now he's starting school for the first time, the staff all have to know exactly how to cope with a reaction if it occurs.

A local charity sponsored Sam to have a Medic Alert bracelet, and this has been of great comfort. We have also ensured that the school staff are kept fully informed about Sam's allergy.

Susie's story

I've known since I was a child that I'm allergic to walnuts – and usually I avoid them like the plague. But last December I was out with my flatmates, Clare and Karen, and I dropped my guard. We were all tasting each other's food and, seconds after taking a forkful of Clare's pasta, my lip began to swell and my tongue started tingling. I knew there were no walnuts in the pasta, but I suddenly realised that on the other side of Clare's plate was something that looked suspiciously like Waldorf salad. My last experience of walnuts was when I ate a Waldorf salad about three years ago. That time I'd made myself sick to try and prevent the reaction, but it didn't work and I'd had to go to the doctor for emergency treatment.

I knew the tingling and swelling around my mouth were just the tip of the iceberg and that the symptoms were probably going to get worse. But I was totally unprepared for how much worse they would become – or how rapidly.

My parents had the tablets I needed, so I phoned and asked them to meet me back at my flat – and my friends and I jumped in a taxi. My body was itching all over and I was wheezing like a heavy smoker. Back home I thought a shower would calm me down. But when Karen and Clare came into the bathroom to check I was OK, I'd collapsed on the floor and was almost unconscious.

Mum and Dad arrived at about the same time and Mum took

one look at me and called an ambulance. Dad tried to give me my tablet. But I couldn't sit up or swallow it, and they were so worried they drove me straight to casualty themselves. I was immediately put on a drip and an oxygen machine and given an injection of adrenaline. And within ten minutes I was beginning to feel a bit better.

Nobody told me what would have happened if I hadn't got to the hospital when I did. But Mum and Dad said they and the casualty team were all very worried about me.

It's not always possible to get a full rundown of every ingredient on a restaurant menu, but I will always question waiters very directly in future. I now have to carry adrenaline wherever I go. It could save my life if I eat the wrong thing.

Susie is very lucky to have got to casualty in time. She accepts now that she must do things differently in order to protect herself. She doesn't taste food unless she knows what is in it. She now carries adrenaline with her at all times. And she has drawn up a crisis plan, under which someone would dial 999 at a very early stage. It could save her life.

- Try to avoid the indiscriminate use of nuts, e.g. powdered nuts as a garnish, unless they're an essential part of a recipe.
- If a dish is meant to contain nuts, why not make sure this is reflected in the name: e.g. nut and carrot salad.
- If possible, keep certain preparation areas designated as nut-free.
- Put up a prominent sign encouraging people with allergies to question staff.
- Include a prominent statement on the menu encouraging customers with severe allergies to question staff. For example: 'Some of our dishes contain nuts. If you are allergic to nuts, please ask the waiter to suggest a nut-free meal.'
- Try to ensure that where a dish contains potent allergens – particularly nuts – this is indicated in some way on the menu. Some restaurants adopt a circled N.
- Organize for your staff a training session on allergies. Make sure that all new staff members (including part-time and casual staff) are aware of serious allergies.

In addition, the Anaphylaxis Campaign offers this advice for waiting staff.

- If a customer claims to have a life-threatening food allergy (anaphylaxis), take the customer seriously. Peanuts and tree nuts are the foods most commonly implicated. But on rare occasions other foods may be mentioned – for example, sesame seeds and other seeds, dairy products, eggs, soya, shellfish, fish, pulses and fresh fruit.
- Find out which member of staff has access to accurate information about ingredients. Approach that person if you need information.
- If there is any serious doubt about whether a food is free of a certain ingredient, such as nuts, admit to the customer that you are unsure.
- If, on examining their meal, a customer realizes it contains nuts and asks you to replace it, remember it is not enough simply to pick the nuts from the plate and return it to the customer. Tiny traces that remain may be enough to cause a severe allergic reaction.
- If there is a gateau covered in nuts on the sweet trolley, ensure that no nuts could possibly be transferred to adjacent sweets.

For all staff, the Anaphylaxis Campaign makes the following points.

- Remember that cooking in unrefined groundnut oil (peanut oil) may leave traces of nut protein in the food being cooked.

- Any oil that has previously been used to cook products containing nuts may contain minute traces of nut proteins.
- If you are preparing food for someone with a severe allergy, beware of transferring food from one dish to another.
- Remember that salad oil may be derived from nut oil.
- Hands, utensils, cutlery and work surfaces should be washed scrupulously after handling foods containing potent allergens.

The Anaphylaxis Campaign has received a batch of letters from happy nut-allergy sufferers who have found and recommended restaurants where allergies are taken into account. One restaurant offered a booklet itemizing the ingredients of every dish on the menu. Another offered to fax over a list of suitable dishes prior to the visit to the restaurant.

It has to be said that other restaurants have been sued by people who have suffered allergic reactions after eating food they were assured was nut free. But, the message seems to be filtering through, and with luck eating out in the future will not be the nightmare for nut allergy sufferers it has been in the past.

The art of self-defence

Avoidance of the culprit foods is an important aspect of allergy management. But accidental exposures do occasionally happen, and so getting top-quality medical guidance is also vital.

In 1994 the Chief Medical Officer told GPs in a bulletin: 'All patients suspected to suffer from peanut allergy should be referred to a specialist clinic. Even if the diagnosis is in doubt, patients should on no account be advised to test their reaction by eating peanuts.' A referral is important for anyone whose symptoms suggest anaphylaxis, whatever the cause.

So anyone who suspects they may be allergic to nuts should go to their GP and seek a referral to an allergy clinic. In that way, a proper assessment of your allergy can be undertaken by an expert. If it is considered that you should be prescribed injectable adrenaline, it is essential to carry it around at all times. Almost all the known deaths attributed to food-related allergic reactions have occurred when adrenaline was not available at an early stage of the reaction.

Make sure you are completely comfortable with both the adrenaline kit and the method of administering it. Make sure everyone in your family knows how to administer it – and when. Do not be frightened of adrenaline. The dose you will administer has very few side-effects, which will pass quickly in any case.

It is important to develop a crisis plan for how to handle an emergency. Get your allergist or GP to help. Have this written out for family and friends – put it on the bulletin board at home; carry one in your pocket. If a child is the person at risk, make sure his teachers and friends' parents have a copy. Make sure everyone knows where the adrenaline is when you go out, or when you are at home.

Coping emotionally

The psychological aspects of anaphylaxis have not been publicized as well as the physical features. However, there are inescapable emotional consequences of a severe nut allergy. Anyone who has experienced an acute attack may have felt close to death. Having had this experience, you may suffer ongoing anxiety, reliving the attack in your mind, and trying to avoid any reminder of it. In the worst scenario this anxiety can interfere with your life, causing difficulty in concentrating, and making you hypervigilant – obsessively aware of everything happening around you. Some people may need professional help to overcome these feelings.

A more dangerous psychological problem to arise from anaphylaxis is denial. You may be so keen to drive the memory of a severe attack from your mind that you block it out completely, refusing to acknowledge that you need to carry your adrenaline with you, and failing to take the usual precautions about foods. Denial enables you to build a protective façade that allows you to continue with your life in a relatively normal way. But you need to understand that you are putting your life at risk if you knowingly expose yourself to nuts.

Teenagers are most at risk from denial. Having avoided an attack for two or three years, they are capable of convincing themselves nothing bad can happen to them. This, coupled with the fact that most teenagers want to be able to lead a normal social life (which involves going to pubs, parties, and Chinese and Indian restaurants – all of which tend to have nuts somewhere to be found), means that, sadly, teenagers with nut allergy are the most likely group to suffer from a potentially fatal allergic reaction. They are too old for their parents to control what they do, and where they go, yet too young to take full control of their own lives.

David Reading, one of the founders of the Anaphylaxis Campaign and father of Sarah, who died in 1993, reported in the British

Allergy Foundation's magazine, *Allergy-Free*, the case of Samantha, a typical teenager with a casual attitude to her allergy.

Samantha started to feel wheezy towards the end of a Christmas party. Her nose and eyes were streaming and she felt a need to sit down. A few minutes later she was having difficulty swallowing – and realized she was having the start of an allergic reaction. She had left her adrenaline at home, having become complacent about the need to carry it. She hadn't needed it for over three years. She was embarrassed about leaving the party, but, when she explained to her host what was happening, her friend agreed to run her to hospital. In casualty she was given prompt treatment and kept in overnight, but was fine the next morning.

It transpired that the party host had placed bowls of peanuts around the room for his guests. It seems likely that the protein from the nuts was transferred to guests' hands on to surfaces such as tables, chairs and beer glasses, and Samantha picked up traces on her own hand and touched her mouth. Because Samantha was in denial about her allergy, she had not registered the danger that the peanuts presented.

Embarrassment is another stumbling block for teenagers. Natalie, a teenager with nut and latex allergies, explains:

'When people think of nut allergy, they think it's dangerous, but they don't think of the embarrassment it can cause. Whenever I eat out with friends, I always have to make a point of asking the waiter if the dish I've chosen contains nuts. If people don't know about my allergy, they think I'm just being difficult.

'If a group of friends suggest going for an Indian meal, I make excuses and leave, because I can't risk eating Indian food – and I'm too embarrassed to have to explain why.'

As a teenager, nut allergy can be excruciatingly embarrassing. You must even remember to check whether someone you're kissing has been eating nuts.

If problems do become unbearable, or you find yourself (or a loved one with an allergy) becoming withdrawn, do consider the help available. Your GP will be able to refer you to a counsellor or behavioural psychotherapist. However, in the vast majority of cases high-quality information is all that is needed so that you are able to take control of your allergy.

Airline travel

Some people with peanut allergy report that they experience symptoms while travelling on aircraft. Often the cause is the free peanut snacks handed around to passengers with their drinks. Once the packets are opened, the peanut dust erupts into the air and is circulated around the aircraft cabin. Symptoms reported include streaming eyes and wheezing. Not every person with peanut allergy reports having this problem, but when it does occur it is extremely distressing.

In response to concerns, some airlines no longer serve peanut snacks, and some will remove them from specified flights if contacted well in advance by the customer. The Anaphylaxis Campaign offers written guidance on this.

For people who suffer severe allergic reactions to food, airline meals may pose a particular risk. Many airlines will organize a special meal according to individual requirements, but mistakes can sometimes occur. Even when an airline has promised a meal free from a certain ingredient, it is important to ensure the information has been passed on down the line. Enquire while checking in, and when boarding the plane. The best advice is to take your own food.

Medic Alert

Although you should always carry your medicine with you, and should always remember your crisis plan, it may be helpful – and reassuring – to know that medics will be able to recognize your problem for what it is if, for any reason, you are unable to explain. The organization Medic Alert is an internationally recognized medical identification system which communicates all your special medical needs quickly and accurately when and where it counts. By wearing a Medic Alert emblem, you will be carrying basic information about yourself and your allergy wherever you go. The emblem also bears Medic Alert's 24-hour emergency number, giving doctors instant access to further information about your allergy. For details see Useful Addresses.

Jane's story

Thirteen years ago my daughter Natalie had her first peanut butter sandwich and her first anaphylactic reaction. During the next few months she had two more reactions. Looking back, they were all quite severe but at that time the only medical advice was: 'Yes, she probably is allergic to nuts – don't give them to her.'

For the next eight years that worked well. But there was never any mention of referral to an allergy clinic or of adrenaline. Then, when we were on holiday in Somerset, Natalie ordered a trifle from a café, having asked if there were nuts on it. There weren't any nuts on it – but they were in it! Within two minutes her throat was closing up and she suffered a major anaphylactic reaction. Fortunately we got her to hospital in time. Our GP referred us to an allergy specialist and we were prescribed an adrenaline injection.

Natalie is now 14 and very aware of her problems but it only makes her more determined to have a normal life and be the best at everything she attempts. She does not like sympathy and will not accept that she is any different from her friends. She is a better reader from reading all those food labels from a very young age! She is a strong swimmer from all that practice to strengthen her lungs (because of her asthma). And she is one of the best cross-country runners in her school year, again thanks to the training to improve her breathing.

As she got older I encouraged her to manage her own medicines and diet. She does this admirably, always taking her 'Thingy' – the affectionately named injector pen – wherever she goes. She has been on a Brownie pack holiday, on residential school trips since the age of nine, away to Guide camp, on canal boat weekends and climbing in the Peak District.

She still enjoys sport and rides her horse four or five times a week as well as training to be a proficient climber. She is learning the saxophone and appears in school plays.

So is her allergy a major problem? Not really. Thanks to her healthy diet she has more energy than most of her friends and due to her determination she meets all life's challenges. Of course, everything she does takes more planning and preparation but I am more than happy to support her. I now have a well-adjusted teenage daughter who makes me extremely proud.

Cosmetics

Nut oils are used in some soaps and cosmetics, but the potential risk these pose for people with nut allergy is not clear.

The good news is that all soaps, cosmetics and personal care products now have to carry full ingredient lists, under a European directive which came into force on 1 January 1999. The bad news is that the ingredients are printed in Latin. This may be perplexing but the European Commission insists this is necessary to standardize the wording.

Apart from soap and cosmetics, products included under the directive are toiletries, perfumes, toothpaste, shampoo, hair care products, creams and deodorants. Without a little knowledge of Latin, if you are looking for allergenic ingredients you will have no idea what words to watch out for.

The Anaphylaxis Campaign believes serious allergic reactions to soaps, shampoos, cosmetics and other personal care products are rare, but you may wish to be aware of these Latin translations:

- Peanut oil: *Arachis oil*
- Bitter almond: *Prunus amara*
- Sweet almond: *Prunus dulcis*
- Sesame: *Sesamum indicum*
- Walnut: *Juglans regia or juglans nigra*
- Brazil: *Bertholletia excelsa*
- Hazelnut: *Corylus rostrata* or *Corylus Americana* or *Corylus avellana*

5

Troubleshooting

Q A large number of foods in my local supermarket now carry warning labels stating, 'may contain nut traces'. Is it safe for me to eat these or not?

A These labels may seem overcautious but they are designed to cover any potential risk if a food not containing nuts has travelled on a conveyor belt previously used for something with nuts in it. Some allergy sufferers have started to voice concerns that extensive labelling by food producers may be simply a legal device, to defend the producer from any action resulting from an accident with their food. The risk then is that sufferers become so complacent they start to eat foods which they should not. Guidelines have been issued by several food industry bodies which aim to minimize risk and reduce the need for 'may contain' labels, and we should see some reduction in so-called defensive labelling in the future. The Anaphylaxis Campaign is pressing for all sections of the food industry to remove altogether – wherever possible – the risk of cross-contamination.

Q I have heard pregnant women are advised to avoid eating peanuts. Why is this?

A This advice from the Department of Health is directed at women who are 'atopic' (prone to allergies such as asthma, eczema or hay fever), and those who have a partner or a child who is atopic. The risk of peanut allergy developing in atopic families is higher than for non-atopic families and there is evidence that peanut proteins can be passed by the mother to the unborn child, sensitizing the baby in the womb. However, more research is needed before the mechanisms of sensitization are fully understood and crystal-clear advice can be provided. At present, the view of the Anaphylaxis Campaign is that women in atopic families should indeed try to avoid peanuts while pregnant, but that avoidance should not become fanatical to the extent that they worry about every 'may contain' warning.

Q Will breastfeeding my baby make her less likely to develop a peanut allergy?

A Breastfed babies are less inclined than bottle-fed infants to develop allergies and asthma, and breastfeeding for at least the first four months (when babies are most susceptible) is always recommended. On the subject of nut allergy, the Department of Health advice is similar to that given to pregnant women: if your immediate family has a strong history of allergic conditions, you 'may wish' to avoid peanuts while breastfeeding. Again, more research is needed here.

Q My son had an allergic reaction to peanut butter when he was nine months old. He's now two years old and my GP has suggested trying him out on a small amount of peanut butter to see if the allergy really is there. Is this safe?

A Allergy to peanuts often remains a lifelong problem, but a few children do grow out of it. Continue to exclude peanuts from your son's diet, and if you want to find out if he's still allergic in the future, ask your GP about getting him tested at an NHS allergy clinic. If the result is inconclusive, a 'challenge test' may be offered. This must be done in hospital – not at home.

Q My toddler has had severe reactions to peanuts. He is due to start nursery school soon. How can I prevent him from coming into contact with peanuts there?

A The first step is to arrange to see the supervisor of your son's nursery school. You must convince him or her of the seriousness of your son's allergy, and the importance of him avoiding peanuts. Explain that peanut allergy can be life-threatening, but it is most certainly manageable. Ask if it would be possible for your son to be closely watched at mealtimes so he does not encounter peanuts. There may be peanuts in another child's packed lunch, so awareness and vigilance among staff and other parents is vital.

The Anaphylaxis Campaign publishes a leaflet called *Anaphylaxis: Guidance for Carers of Pre-School Children*. Give a copy of this to the nursery school. In it the Campaign explains what anaphylaxis is, and how teachers can draw up a management plan to cover contact details, emergency procedure, medication and precautionary measures.

Q Are there any special guidelines for schools on the management of a nut allergy?

A Research suggests that at least one child in every school may have peanut allergy. In many cases it is potentially serious. This is understandably alarming for teachers and other school staff. However, the vast majority of these children are in mainstream schools, and, with sound precautionary measures and support from

31

the staff, school life may continue as normal for all concerned. The Anaphylaxis Campaign's booklet, *Anaphylaxis and Schools: How We Can Make It Work*, offers invaluable help.

Schools need to draw up a policy for day-to-day management of the child's allergy to cover food preparation, school outings, and craft, cookery and science classes which may use nut ingredients. There should also be an emergency action plan in force, and an individual protocol for each allergic child should be drawn up.

It will also be useful to get hold of the DfEE/DoH document entitled *Supporting pupils with medical needs in schools*. This is available from DfEE Publications, PO Box 5050, Sherwood Park, Annesley, Nottinghamshire NG15 0DJ (tel. 0845 6022260).

Q I suffer with swelling of the lips and tingling in my mouth whenever I eat nuts. I have heard that avoiding them for a year will get rid of my allergy. Is this true?

A Unfortunately not. Nut allergy is usually a lifelong condition. But not every case is serious. You need to get your allergy properly assessed at an NHS allergy clinic.

Q I've been told that the peanut is not actually a nut, but a legume – so why must I avoid other nuts if I am only allergic to peanuts?

A One reason is that peanuts are sometimes used as a cheap substitute for more expensive nuts as they can be made to taste like almonds, walnuts or brazil nuts. A survey in the West Country a few years ago showed that almond slices sold in some bakery shops in fact contained peanuts instead of almonds. There is also the risk that peanuts may be 'contaminated' with traces of other nuts. So the advice is often given that people with peanut allergy should play safe and avoid all nut products.

Q How safe are the skin-prick tests to identify allergies? I suffered a severe reaction to something I ate but I don't know exactly what the culprit was. My GP has suggested I get tested – but I'm nervous of this.

A Each year 10 per cent of the UK population experiences an allergic problem of some kind, and 25 per cent of the population will, during their lifetimes, see a doctor because of an allergy. As these problems are now so common, allergy testing is being carried out more often and is becoming increasingly sophisticated. But every test has its advantages and disadvantages. Skin-prick testing is usually the first to be suggested. You may have to give up certain medicines for a period before the test is carried out, and this should only be done under the guidance of your doctor. The test may show reactions to substances which do not at present cause symptoms. These results may indicate a latent allergy which could become a problem later in life. The test is simple, quick and inexpensive, providing results within 15 minutes. If you have previously suffered a severe anaphylactic shock, there is a small risk that the skin test will cause a similar reaction. This is very rare, but must be discussed with your GP. Even in the unlikely event that you had a severe reaction to a test, the person testing you will have all the resources needed to treat the reaction immediately, so you will come to no harm.

Q My son is allergic to peanuts. Does this mean he can't eat other members of the legume family?

A An American study found that 5 per cent of their selected population of children who reacted to legumes suffered symptoms with multiple legumes. People with peanut allergy need to be aware of this possibility. But it is probably unnecessary to eliminate other legumes (such as peas, beans and lentils) from the diet unless there is good reason to suspect they cause problems.

Q How can I be sure I won't be served foods containing peanut while I'm on holiday?

A Unless you want a completely self-catering holiday (fresh food and all, so you don't encounter any unidentifiable ingredients), you will have to explain your allergy to the people serving and cooking your food. If you're not fluent in the language of the country where you're staying, take a pre-written card. The British Allergy Foundation produces a series of cards in various languages. But be prepared for accidents, as always. Carry your adrenaline with you at all times and be extra safe by wearing a Medic Alert emblem. The Anaphylaxis Campaign provides written guidance, on request, for people flying off on holiday.

Q My best friend has asthma, which is well controlled by her medication. Why is my allergy to sesame seeds not controllable in the same way?

A Food allergies cannot be controlled in the same way as asthma. The only way you can keep yourself safe is to avoid eating sesame seeds. Desensitization, also known as immunotherapy, is available for some allergies, such as insect venom allergy. It involves a series of injections of very small amounts of an allergen over a long period.

The idea is gradually to build up your immune system's tolerance to the substance you're allergic to. But you should be very wary of anyone offering desensitization to severe food allergy.

Q My son recently had a terrible anaphylactic reaction to food containing peanuts. Why did it affect his whole body, and not just his mouth and stomach?

A Your son's body produced a large number of chemical substances in response to the peanut allergen, and these were spread around his body by his bloodstream, causing swelling and leaking of blood vessels. In the lungs this causes wheezing and breathing difficulties. In the bowels it causes nausea and stomach cramps. All the organs of the body can be affected differently by anaphylaxis. As fluid leaks out of the small blood vessels, the total volume of blood in the body is reduced, and this means blood pressure drops and the heart has trouble pumping hard enough to get blood to the vital organs. Very quickly, you can become dizzy or faint, or even fall unconscious. The sooner treatment is given, the better.

Q How do I know if I'm at risk of anaphylactic shock?

A Unfortunately there's no way of knowing for sure until you have an attack. People with a history of allergic conditions (e.g. asthma, hay fever and eczema) are more at risk, and nut allergy can be particularly severe in some cases. However, full-blown anaphylactic shock is quite rare. In all cases the message is this: have your allergy properly assessed at an NHS allergy clinic and carry prescribed medication at all times.

Q My son has been prescribed an adrenaline auto-injector, but I'm unclear about how to use it. How can I find out?

A The adrenaline comes with instructions, and it's important to familiarize yourself with these before an emergency arises. If there's anything you don't understand, discuss this with your GP or practice nurse, and refresh your memory by reading the instructions every month or so. The Anaphylaxis Campaign has produced a useful video for schools which covers the administering of adrenaline.

Q My daughter has had three moderately bad allergic reactions to peanuts and carries an adrenaline injector. But we're not sure at what stage during a reaction it should be administered.

A This is a difficult one, because each reaction may present differently and not every reaction needs adrenaline. Anyone who has suffered full-blown anaphylactic shock in the past certainly needs to be aware that any future reaction might be severe, and should be ready to administer adrenaline. Even mild or moderate symptoms can be followed by more severe ones at a later date, although this is not always the case.

Your daughter's individual case should be discussed with a health professional, but there are some general guidelines. Watch the symptoms carefully. Is there a marked difficulty in breathing or swallowing? Is there sudden weakness or floppiness? Is there a steady deterioration? Any of these are signs of a serious reaction. Administer adrenaline without delay if you believe the symptoms are serious, or becoming serious. If in any doubt at all, give the adrenaline.

It is important to work out a written crisis plan in advance, with the help of your doctor, and ensure that anyone looking after your daughter has a copy.

It must also be remembered that when a reaction occurs, an ambulance must be called and ambulance control needs to be told that it is a suspected case of anaphylaxis. A second injection of adrenaline may be given after five–ten minutes if the ambulance hasn't arrived and there is no improvement.

Q Is adrenaline ever dangerous to use?

A Adrenaline has been used for over 100 years and is well understood and very reliable. Unless you are very elderly or have a heart condition, there is no need to worry about using it. All it will do is push your heart rate up to the sort of level it would reach if you had just been playing sport. But adrenaline can be dangerous if given directly into a vein. The injection you are prescribed must be administered in the side of the thigh, which is perfectly safe.

Q I am allergic to walnuts and have now had tests which reveal I'm also allergic to almonds. Are the two nuts related?

A It's quite common for people to be allergic to both walnuts and almonds as the nuts have chemical similarities. Pistachios and cashews are also chemically alike, and some people are allergic to both of these. It's sensible for people with nut allergy to play safe and avoid all nuts.

Q I'm sure eating peanuts makes my asthma worse, but my GP seems sceptical about this link.

A Any food can cause asthma, with the symptoms normally coming on within hours. You should ask your GP to refer you to an allergy specialist so that an expert's view can be obtained. Ensure that you always use your asthma drugs to prevent an attack (see Chapter 6).

Q My eczema is always worse under stress, and I have been considering booking a course of massages to help myself relax. However, I am scared the oil the masseuse uses may trigger an allergic reaction, as I react to nuts. What should I do?

A Explain your problem to the masseuse, and she will be careful to select a base oil that does not contain almond for your massage. Certain aromatherapy oils can help eczema, so as well as helping you relax, the treatment should be beneficial for your skin.

Q Can complementary medicine help my peanut allergy?

A Complementary medicine means just that – it should be used alongside orthodox medicine, rather than instead of it. Acupuncture, acupressure and homeopathy may all be helpful for asthma (alongside conventional treatment), and Chinese herbalism, and naturopathy may help eczema. It would, however, be unwise to trust a complementary therapy to treat a severe allergy to nuts, in which case emergency treatment with adrenaline as described throughout this book is really the only answer to a severe allergic reaction.

Q Could cot death be due to anaphylaxis?

A Cases of cot death have fallen since parents have been advised to put their babies on their backs to sleep, instead of their fronts. But the cause for the remaining deaths is still unknown. Allergy may be a factor, and this is one area being researched.

Q I've heard that anaphylaxis can be mistaken for a heart attack. Why is this?

A Usually a heart attack is heralded by severe chest pain – but occasionally there is very little warning before the sufferer collapses, which is why anaphylaxis can be mistaken for a heart attack. Another cause of confusion is the fact that both emergencies can be accompanied by stomach pain. The key is to be aware of the symptoms of anaphylaxis (see p. 13), and to know who is likely to suffer an attack.

6

Other Allergic Conditions

It is common for people with nut allergy to have other allergic conditions, such as asthma, eczema and hay fever. Therefore, although this book is about nut allergy, it is appropriate to look at some of these other complaints. Their proper management forms an important part of an overall strategy.

Asthma

There has been a fourfold increase in the numbers of children suffering from asthma over the last 20 years. Asthma is now the commonest reason for children to be admitted to hospital and in many areas is one of the leading causes of admissions for adults as well.

Most – but not all – people who suffer from severe food allergies also have asthma. And for these people, asthma is a significant risk factor. During a severe allergic reaction, asthma can be one of the main features and one of the most serious ones. Good day-by-day control of asthma is believed to lower the risk of an allergic reaction being life-threatening.

If someone has an immediate food allergy and chronic allergic asthma, management of allergic reactions should include antihistamine, asthma reliever medications and injectable adrenaline. Management of the food allergy should also focus on reducing allergens from the home environment, such as house dust mite or cat.

Allergy-induced asthma is more likely to occur in people who have other allergic conditions such as hay fever, and in those whose asthma is also triggered by, for example, dust, pollens and animals. And it's worth bearing in mind that asthma triggered by a food allergy may take several hours to develop, and so food might not be identified as the cause. It is possible that unexplained bouts of asthma may be caused, in some cases, by inadvertent exposure to a food, such as nuts, cows' milk, egg or fish.

The fact that asthma is difficult to diagnose in very young children makes many parents worry that GPs are becoming 'steroid-happy', prescribing aerosol puffer drugs at the first hint of a wheeze. If anything, surveys show that doctors are still under-diagnosing slightly. It's reassuring that these drugs have been around for a quarter of a century and are well understood. Most prominent allergy experts in the UK are convinced that they are an important weapon in the fight against asthma and, moreover, that they reduce the risk of severe allergic reactions for those who are prone to them.

It is also becoming clear that children with allergies and asthma may face an increased risk of a bad reaction if their parents smoke. Breathing in cigarette smoke may impair the lungs and raise the risk of severe asthma in the event of a reaction to the food or substance to which they are allergic. Parents who smoke may also increase the risk of an allergy developing in their children in the first place. Many doctors believe it should be standard advice to parents of allergic children not to smoke. This advice should be given as early as possible to families in which there is a history of allergies – preferably at pre-conception stage and certainly during pregnancy.

Other factors may play a part in the current asthma epidemic:

- Air pollution – so far, there's no proof that this is behind the increase in numbers of sufferers. But it does worsen asthma for established sufferers.
- The way we live – for example more of us have double glazing, central heating and fitted carpets, and this warmer, more humid environment is the perfect breeding ground for the number one asthma trigger – the house dust mite.
- The modern diet – eating more processed foods and fewer fresh foods – may affect the development of children's immune systems, making them more susceptible to conditions like asthma.
- How well mothers look after themselves in pregnancy. Smoking in pregnancy has already been shown to make children more susceptible to asthma. Now experts think it's also likely that mothers who lack important nutrients in their diet during pregnancy are putting their babies at increased risk of developing asthma.

Finally, although it is important to follow your doctor's advice relating to good asthma control, some practitioners believe there is also value in some additional methods to improve breathing. These include:

- Buteyko – a system of breathing exercises intended to alter the balance of oxygen and carbon dioxide in exhaled air. Those who practise the technique believe that people with asthma (and many other conditions) 'over-breathe' and, by doing so, lose too much carbon dioxide from their system. Many patients who have tried the method report positive results. But the National Asthma Campaign says research is needed to prove its value, including detailed studies exploring the long-term effects of the technique. Before starting a Buteyko course it is essential to discuss this with your doctor and you should be careful to keep up your preventer drugs throughout.

- Powerbreathe – a hand-held device with a tube to the mouth through which you breathe in order to exercise and strengthen the lungs. The device is also used for older people who suffer with shortness of breath, and, in tests, asthma sufferers were 12.4 per cent less breathless during exercise.

About asthma

- Asthma is a condition which causes difficulty in moving air into and out of the lungs as we breathe. The main components are bronchospasm, inflammation of the lining of the airways and excessive mucus.

- Symptoms include coughing, chest tightness, wheezing and shortness of breath. You may also have tightness in your chest, sharp chest pains and, more rarely, itchy or tingly skin.

- Triggers which bring on these symptoms include:
  – colds and viruses
  – exercise
  – stress
  – changes in the weather
  – cigarette smoke
  – allergies, especially the house dust mite. Nuts may be a problem if some of these other conditions already apply.
  – drugs, e.g. aspirin, Nurofen, ibuprofen, and beta-blockers used for high blood pressure and heart problems.

- The cause of asthma is often an inherited tendency. Most often this comes out in childhood, but the first symptoms can be much later in life.

- Asthma can't be cured, but with careful control, using inhaled steroids, you can lead a normal life.

Alison's story

I always used to think that asthma was something sickly little children had – not a condition you could develop in adulthood.

But, four years ago, I started getting bouts of eczema, and, after two years, my GP sent me to an allergy clinic for tests. There I discovered I was allergic to the house dust mite and pets – both of which are also well-known triggers for asthma. So when I first became wheezy, the following Christmas, it wasn't a huge surprise.

We'd spent Christmas with my parents, who have two cats. My eczema was really flaring up around then, and I was also quite run-down with a very bad cold.

By the time we got home, I was beginning to wheeze – but I put it down to my cold and didn't think too much about it. Then, a couple of weeks later, I found myself struggling for breath when I climbed the stairs or walked in the park with my children, Josh, four, and Nina, two.

My partner, John, was working away, and I was finding it difficult to cope with everyday activities because my chest was so tight. I couldn't push the buggy without stopping every few yards for a rest – but I only finally realized how bad I was when, staying over at my brother's, I had to stop half-way up the stairs and sit down for a few seconds because I couldn't go any further.

Luckily I had booked an appointment with my GP for the next day as I was due to see her about my eczema. So I told her all about my wheeziness, and, after getting me to breathe into a monitor, she told me I definitely had asthma.

My first thought was of the asthmatic children I used to go to school with. They were always the ones who couldn't take part in sports, and I thought, 'Goodness, I'm not going to be able to do anything!' We were about to go on holiday for a week, and I'd been looking forward to cycling with the children and joining in aerobics sessions. I didn't want to be a miserable invalid, stuck on my own in the lodge while John played with the children.

The doctor reassured me that, in fact, doing these sports would be no problem – as long as I took the medicines she was about to give me. It seems I had a pretty old-fashioned idea of what asthma is. These days it doesn't affect sufferers' lives to the extent that it used to.

My GP gave me two inhalers: one containing salbutamol,

which I had to take two puffs from four times a day, and one containing beclomethasone 100 which I was to use first thing in the morning and last thing at night.

She showed me how to use the puffers (there's quite a knack to it), and said that I was bound to feel the difference within a few days. Happily, she was right about that – a week later, I'd improved so much that the holiday was no problem for me.

After my asthma diagnosis, I came away from the surgery with a costly list of prescription medicines. But despite my initial fears about the regular expenses I'd soon be running up, I was so much better within a month that I no longer had to use my treatments.

I've had no bad attacks since then, but I'm aware of the need to prevent these by keeping the house as dust-free as possible. My diagnosis coincided with a move to a new house. So this was the perfect opportunity to start afresh with bare floorboards, frequent vacuuming, and keeping soft toys and clothes shut away in cupboards instead of lying around where they can collect dust. I'm told these simple measures can make a big difference to asthma – so it's silly not to take them.

Eczema

The word eczema comes from ancient Greek and literally means 'to boil over' – which is just what sufferers feel their skin is doing as it becomes itchy, hot and inflamed.

One in ten of us suffers to some degree (one in 12 adults and one in eight children) and the condition can start at any age.

There is no single cure for eczema, but in most cases it can be kept at bay using prescribed treatments.

Research shows that babies with atopic eczema have a 70 per cent chance of developing asthma.

Stress, skin contact with chemicals, soap or perfume are common triggers, and food allergy can also play a big part, as the story of Joe illustrates below. Joe's case is at the extreme end of the spectrum but, thankfully, his family have learned how to cope with his eczema.

Joe's story

Joe's skin was perfect until he started on solid food, when he developed angry patches on his cheeks, chin and folds of his neck. His GP gave him some cream but the eczema kept on

41

spreading – affecting the crooks of the arms, backs of the knees and around the ankles. His thumbs, which he sucked a lot, became cracked open and weeping. He was given antihistamines and steroid creams, but these didn't help him sleep any better at night, so by this time he was crabby all day as well as all night. The whole family was being kept awake by his crying and scratching. Worst of all, whenever he got a cold he would wipe his nose with those cracked, raw fingers and inevitably began to get nasty infections.

On one occasion he was taken to the A&E department of the local hospital as blisters spread up his arm from a hand infection and his temperature shot up. The next day he screamed with pain as it took two nurses to hold him down as his saturated dressing was changed.

The worst times of all for itching were when he had to get undressed for anything, when he got really hot, or when he was stressed. Eczema is such a horrible and vicious circle – it itches so you scratch, but when you scratch it makes it worse, and when it does begin to get better it itches again, so you scratch and make it worse again.

When his skin was bad, one of the worst things was having a bath. Every day his mother would run him a bath. Joe would stand in the bath and cry. Getting his skin wet hurt so much.

His parents were getting desperate, and asked their GP for a referral to a specialist. Joe had developed asthma as well. With dashes to the hospital for the nebulizer, treating skin infections, sleepless nights from scratching and wheezing, on top of the normal mishaps any adventurous toddler undergoes, his mother was exhausted.

A blood test revealed that Joe's eczema was an allergic reaction to eggs. His mother was horrified! She had been feeding him eggs most days since he had been weaned on to solids, and had no idea they were the cause of his skin problems. But even after she dropped eggs from Joe's diet, the eczema persisted. In fact, they discovered much later that he was allergic to a number of different foods and additives.

On the first visit to the skin specialist Joe was put in wet-wraps and prescribed evening primrose oil. The specialist explained how eczema could react to factors in the environment. He recommended that Joe's parents find out as much as they could about eczema, so that they would be better equipped to deal with his skin. They were told about an organization called the National Eczema Society which would provide them with information and advice. 'We joined up – sending for all the leaflets we could get hold of.'

So began a process of learning which continues to this day. From that moment Joe's mother and father began to take control of his eczema instead of letting it control all of them. Joe's mother learnt how to apply the wet-wraps herself. The ones the nurse had applied stayed in place for days, and when his mother took them off again Joe's skin was baby-soft, if marked by lingering red patches. Her own first attempts resulted in her child looking like a mummy from a horror film – loops of steroid-stained gauze unravelling within hours of being so laboriously applied. But gradually her bandaging skills improved and Joe grew to love the comfort that they brought him.

She studied all the information that the National Eczema Society sent and as she discovered what kinds of things contributed to Joe's eczema, tried to eliminate them from the home, and especially from his bedroom. She waged war against the pernicious house-dust mite, washing and damp-dusting everything she could, replacing bedding and furnishings with those that could be kept dust-free. She made sure they were all dressed only in cotton, which was washed in non-biological detergents. Joe's usual bath products were stopped and they began, as his father quipped, 'to just give him a wipe over with an oily rag from time to time'. They experimented with different emollients until they found one that suited Joe's skin.

Every small change which was made had a corresponding effect on Joe's skin until the eczema was finally subdued. He is 11 years old now and to look at him you would not guess how hard his parents had to work to look after his skin. It has been a very long haul, but anti-eczema measures have become part of the family routine and are not the burdens they were to begin with. They have all learned to live with eczema.

Types of eczema

- Atopic – which usually starts in childhood and runs in families. It's linked with hay fever and asthma.
- Irritant contact dermatitis – a reaction to substances like detergent, which, if avoided, clears the problem.
- Allergic contact dermatitis – the body mounts an immune

response to certain substances such as nickel, rubber, glue, cosmetics.

- Seborrhoeic eczema – starts as an itchy scalp with severe dandruff and spreads to affect the face and oily areas of the body, especially where there's body hair. Avoiding irritating toiletries can help.
- Pompholyx eczema may occur in combination with atopic or contact eczema. Itchy blisters develop on the sides of the fingers, palms of the hands, and soles of the feet. The skin may dry out and peel and there's a risk of bacterial infection.
- Nummular or discoid eczema – scaly, itchy, coin-shaped patches on the limbs which may blister and weep and become infected.
- Light-sensitive eczema – a rare form of eczema, triggered by sunshine, which may exacerbate another form of eczema.
- Varicose eczema – usually occurs on the lower legs of middle-aged or elderly people. As the skin is thin, it can break down to form varicose ulcers if it is untreated.

Treatments

Although there's no known cure for eczema there is a wide range of treatments available to help control the symptoms. These include:

- Emollients (e.g. Oilatum Bath Formula, or Lotil Original Formula Cream), which are a mixture of oils, fats and water. They restore the moisture content of the skin and break the itch and scratch cycle, giving the skin a chance to recover.
- Topical steroids (e.g. hydrocortisone), which are prescribed for severe cases of eczema but must be used sparingly and under medical guidance as, used long term, they can thin the skin and cause more problems.

  Hydrocortisone can be bought over the counter from chemists but mustn't be used on children under the age of ten, pregnant women, or on the face or genitals, and should never be used for longer than ten days without your GP's permission.
- Antihistamines, which aid sleep and relieve itching.

Hay fever

Also known as allergic rhinitis, hay fever now affects one in five of the population. The causes include pollen, the house dust mite and pets. As you know too well if you are a sufferer, it's not just your nose that is affected. One of the most troublesome symptoms is itchy eyes that water all the time, a condition known as allergic conjunctivitis.

The management of hay fever has been transformed by the fact that you can now buy virtually all the necessary treatments over the counter from the pharmacy without a prescription. You can usually get good advice from your doctor or pharmacist.

It's important to manage hay fever properly because inflammation in the nose and throat can easily track down into the chest causing asthma. Once you have asthma, the symptoms can develop again in the same circumstances.

Perennial rhinitis is basically hay fever symptoms all the year round, usually caused by a range of allergens including dust mite, moulds and animal dander. It is important to treat the symptoms properly as they can lead to asthma.

Urticaria

Also known as hives or nettle rash, urticaria is an itchy skin condition – often short-lived, but not always. It is usually an allergic reaction to something, but it can affect people who are not allergy prone. Allergic causes include bee and wasp stings, foods such as milk, beans, fish, shellfish and nuts, and drugs such as penicillin. Non-allergic causes include cold, heat, water and sunlight; drugs such as paracetamol and aspirin; and certain food dyes and additives. Treatment includes taking regular antihistamines and avoiding the trigger.

As a footnote, the following case is interesting. A child was seen at an allergy clinic who had had several allergic reactions to peanuts. The child had poorly controlled asthma, eczema and rhinitis that improved considerably when the child went on holiday with his family. There was a cat at home and the child had a large positive skin test to cat. After some discussion, the family decided to find another home for the cat. The child's asthma, eczema and rhinitis improved considerably. While he remained allergic to peanut, the child's doctors believe that by removing exposure to other allergens and controlling the child's asthma, his risk for anaphylaxis in the future will be reduced. Ongoing research is being carried out in London to study interactions with asthma, food allergies and rhinitis.

7
Nut-free Nutrition

If you discover you are allergic to nuts, you must avoid them at all costs. Sometimes this is not as easy as it sounds, but if you are committed to remaining vigilant whenever food is around, you can learn to minimize the risks. The key points are:

- Always read food labels scrupulously every time you shop. Even when you buy something you've tried before, read the label. Recipes do sometimes change.
- If in doubt about any product, contact the manufacturer or retailer. Some companies produce lists of their nut-free products. These are extremely useful.
- Look out for 'may contain' warning labels. Normally these appear near the ingredient list, although sometimes they are less easy to spot. Look for them carefully. It's best to take them seriously, even where you suspect they are just a legal device.
- Take particular care if you buy goods from in-store bakeries, because retailers cannot guarantee the absence of nut traces on any product sold there.
- Take particular care, too, when eating out. Most of the severe incidents happen when food is bought in restaurants, hotels, takeaways and other catering outlets. Question staff calmly but directly. If possible, contact them in advance by fax or phone asking if they can ensure you a nut-free meal. If you are in any doubt about their response, try elsewhere.

Next, you must consider whether, by avoiding nuts, you may be missing out on any of the essential nutrients your body needs. This may be true, in particular, if you are a vegetarian. You can always ask your GP to refer you to a registered dietitian, but I hope to provide some useful information here.

While considering your diet, obviously you need to take account of other foods you are allergic to. You may already know what these are – or you may need to undergo testing at an allergy clinic (see Chapter 2).

It is also worth considering whether you have a food intolerance. This is different from an allergy, which is an immune response;

intolerance is triggered by other mechanisms. Whereas food allergy reactions are usually immediate, food intolerance reactions tend to be much slower. The culprits in intolerance are foods that are eaten regularly, especially items such as wheat and milk that are consumed at almost every meal. The slowness of the reaction, combined with the fact that the foods are eaten so often, contributes to the fact that the link between the food and symptoms is often difficult to make. Although food intolerance is not recognized by all doctors, there is a growing body which believes it should be taken seriously. Symptoms might include migraine, fatigue, depression, lethargy, hyperactivity in children, recurrent mouth ulcers, aching muscles, vomiting, nausea, ulcers, diarrhoea, constipation, joint pain and bloating. Of course, if you believe you have a food intolerance it is important to see your doctor so that all possible causes of your symptoms are considered.

As this is a book on nut allergy, I will not explore such a specialized subject as food intolerance, but suggest that those who are interested should read *The Complete Guide to Food Allergy and Intolerance*, by Professor Jonathan Brostoff and Linda Gamlin.

The Mediterranean diet

To stay healthy, many people go for the so-called 'ideal' diet – the Mediterranean diet. This is less about losing weight and more about eating healthily, so you can follow it even if you don't have to lose weight.

- At least 50 per cent of your daily energy should come from complex carbohydrates such as wholegrain rice and pasta and pulses.
- You should eat 400–800 g of fresh fruit and raw or lightly steamed vegetables (not potatoes) per day.
- Fish is rich in essential fatty acids, which help lower harmful blood cholesterol levels. Pulses are also to be recommended – so long as you are not allergic to them!
- Less than 30 per cent of your daily energy should come from fat. Use more olive oil (which should be stored in cool, dark conditions for it to offer the best benefits to your health) and less butter. Eat fish two or three times a week, try to have one or two vegetarian days every week, and try to eat red meat no more than

once or twice a week. Although you don't have to cut out red meat altogether, research shows that a diet of bread, pasta, olive oil, fish, vegetables, fruit, garlic and fresh herbs is beneficial in terms of health.

The best methods for preparing food include:

- eating fruit and vegetables raw or only lightly steamed;
- grilling food with only a light brushing of olive or rapeseed oil;
- baking;
- steaming;
- boiling with only minimal amounts of water and no added salt;
- poaching in vegetable stock;
- stir-frying using a light brushing of olive or rapeseed oil;
- roasting only if the meat is on a rack so the juice and fat runs away;
- making low-fat gravies using granules and the vegetable water instead of the meat juices.

Rules for vegetarians

The Vegetarian Society estimates that there are four million vegetarians in Britain, and 5,000 more are joining their ranks each week. But, unless you are a vegetarian who eats a full and varied range of vegetables, grains and pulses, your diet runs the risk of being nutritionally inadequate.

The key is to make your diet as broad as you can. Most of us settle into a pattern of eating favourite foods over and over again. We may have a set routine with cereal and toast for breakfast, sandwich (choice of two favourite fillings) for lunch, and a pasta or rice based meal for supper. There may be nothing wrong with any of these foods. However, the more you eat something regularly, the more you are in danger of developing a chronic intolerance to it (that is to say the food may be doing you harm without your knowing it). More to the point, you are not allowing yourself to explore a full range of nutrients.

The World Health Organization recommends we eat five portions of fresh fruit and vegetables daily. If possible, eat more – but make variety your goal, choosing as many different vegetables as you can in the course of a week.

This may sound difficult if you're stuck in a rut of peas, broccoli and carrots on the veg side, and apples, bananas and oranges in the way of fruit, but there are many tempting alternatives – roasted sweet potato, parsnip and carrot with stir-fried greens; celeriac and potato mash; braised celery, fennel and leeks. As an exercise, write down as many combinations as you can of four vegetables/fruit you'd like to eat together, without using the same vegetable more than twice. You'll be surprised what you come up with.

Why we need ...

Plenty of fruit and vegetables

They are number one on the list of immune-boosting foods because they're packed with antioxidants which stifle ageing cells. Eat at least five servings a day, and get as much variety as you can (see the box on pages 51–2). Spread them through the day to give your blood a constant flow of antioxidants to fight the free radicals which cause cell damage. If you start young – in childhood – you will prevent much of the cell damage which shows up as premature ageing later in life.

By your thirties and forties, the antioxidant protection of fruit and vegetables is crucial to help you from developing degenerative ageing diseases.

Fish at least two or three times a week

Fatty fish such as salmon, mackerel, sardines, tuna and herring are best as they contain the most omega-3 type fatty acids. These keep the body's cells healthy and intact and also help you to make prostaglandins to keep the body in good running order.

Water

If you are under stress, eat a lot of junk food, and smoke, or take any drugs (including alcohol), you may feel lacking in energy and you may wonder if a vitamin supplement would perk you up. In fact taking unnecessary supplements could just add to the stress and dehydration you're already suffering, because your body will respond by protecting the cell membranes with a shell of cholesterol to keep all the fluids intact inside each cell. If these fluids are trapped inside the cells for too long they become stagnant and toxic, causing more health problems. To rehydrate, we should all aim to drink four pints (two litres) of plain water every day. This helps the body get rid of trapped toxins, and restores normal levels of energy and good health.

Adding more rice, fresh vegetables and pulses to your diet helps with the rehydration process, as well as providing the balance of minerals and vitamins your body needs.

Soya bean foods

Soya milk, soya flour, whole soya beans, tofu, miso and textured soya protein are available in good supermarkets and health food shops. Soya contains many antioxidants and other substances thought to deter certain cancers. But remember that soya is a fairly common allergen. If you believe you may be allergic to it, see your doctor and discuss a referral.

Fewer calories

If you restrict your calories but keep them high quality, so you're lean but not malnourished, you'll dramatically increase your chances of staying young and living longer. Every time you eat something, your body has to process more oxygen to turn that food into energy, and this process triggers the production of harmful free radicals, which damage cells so they age faster. Make every calorie count, and don't squander your allowance on empty foods like sugar. If you're looking to cut down, 1,800 nutritious calories a day is an ideal starting point for an average-sized woman. Don't attempt to lose weight too quickly as this will speed up your ageing process.

Fewer harmful fats

These include:

- meat fat;
- dairy fat (e.g. cream and full-fat cheese);
- polyunsaturated fats;
- partially hydrogenated fats in margarines, vegetable oils and processed foods.

Eat *more* olive oil, which is low in harmful fats.

Less meat

Meat sabotages your cells. But some simple measures, including how you cook it, can help curb the damage if you can't give it up.

- Remove any fat.
- Eat small portions of meat only, with lots of vegetables and rice or pasta.
- Stick to a maximum of three meat-containing dishes a week.
- Boil, stew or poach meat, or cook it in the microwave before grilling, to reduce harmful substances known as HCAs (heterocyclic amines) produced in the cooking process. HCAs are produced when you brown meat, and they stimulate free radicals and cause extensive cell damage.

Fewer sweets

Sugar, cakes and biscuits raise blood insulin levels, damaging arteries and promoting cancer and other degenerative diseases.

More garlic

It's one of the most ancient and respected carriers of antioxidants. Studies in humans and animals suggest it inhibits cancer, artery clogging and degenerative brain function due to ageing. Aim to eat a clove a day, raw or cooked, as a natural anti-ageing medicine. But remember that some people are allergic to it.

Super immune-boosting fruits and vegetables

1 Berries – e.g. strawberries and raspberries – are loaded with antioxidants and save your cells from premature ageing.
2 Broccoli – it's packed with free radical fighters and is one of the richest sources of chromium, a known life extender and protector against the ravages of out-of-control insulin and blood sugar.
3 Cabbage – especially savoy cabbage – is a stomach and breast cancer deterrent. Eat it raw or lightly cooked (stir-fried).

51

4 Carrots – the beta carotene in them is legendary for fighting off disease. One cup of carrot juice contains 24 mg of beta carotene (compared to 6 mg per whole carrot).

5 Citrus fruits – especially grapefruit – are packed with antioxidants.

6 Grapes – especially purple ones – contain powerful antioxidants in their skin and seeds.

7 Onions – which, like garlic, have the ability to bust blood clots and hinder the clogging of arteries.

8 Spinach – cuts the risk of cancer and blindness.

9 Tomatoes – the richest source of the antioxidant lycopene which preserves mental agility.

PART TWO

Recipes

RECIPES

These recipe suggestions are intended mostly to provide some inspiration, especially for vegetarians. If you are prone to allergies though, remember that anything has the potential to cause a problem, so please go carefully. Although I have made these recipes as 'allergy free' as possible, I may have missed your particular trigger.

Special occasion food

Christmas is a time when much of the delicious food which abounds seems to contain nuts. This means that you'll probably need to avoid buying Christmas cakes, mince pies, Christmas puddings and shortbread (often contains almond) and make your own. You can follow any recipe, but substitute the nuts and other problem foods with extra dried fruit to make sure you have the correct proportions of ingredients.

Note: measures are given in both metric and imperial (the conversions are *approximate*, having been rounded up or down). Use either system – not a mixture of the two – in any recipe. All spoon measures are level unless stated otherwise.

STARTERS

Pumpkin soup with cumin and ginger

1 kg/2 lb butternut squash
1 small onion
30 ml/2 tbsp oil
1 heaped tsp cumin
1 heaped tsp grated fresh
  ginger

2 cloves garlic, finely chopped
1.3 litres/2$\frac{1}{4}$ pints vegetable
  stock
salt and pepper to taste

Peel the butternut squash and cut it into chunks. Peel and dice the onion, and sauté it in the oil until transparent. Add the garlic, ginger and cumin and cook for a minute. Add the butternut squash, stir, add stock and simmer until tender (about 30 minutes).

Purée the soup, and add salt and pepper to taste. For a creamier soup, crème fraiche, cream or yogurt can be stirred in before serving.

Garlic soup

Serves 4

16 large cloves garlic,
  unpeeled
900 ml/1$\frac{1}{2}$ pints water
5 ml/1 tsp salt
a little black pepper
5 ml/1 tsp mixed dried herbs

2 cloves
4 sprigs of parsley
3 egg yolks
75 ml/5 tbsp olive oil

Boil the garlic in the water with the salt, pepper, herbs, cloves and parsley for 30 minutes, covered.

Meanwhile, beat the egg yolks in a bowl and stir in the olive oil drop by drop, to make a thick mayonnaise base.

Beat a little of the hot garlic liquid into the egg mixture, and then, very gradually, strain in the rest through a sieve (pressing the juice out of the garlic cloves with a spoon), beating all the time. Serve immediately.

Gazpacho

Serves 4

450 g / 1 lb tomatoes, peeled
a few dice of cucumber
2 cloves garlic, chopped
1 spring onion, finely sliced
12 black olives, stoned
a few strips of green pepper
45 ml / 3 tbsp olive oil
15 ml / 1 tbsp wine vinegar

salt and pepper
a pinch cayenne pepper
a little fresh marjoram, mint,
    or parsley, chopped
300 ml / ½ pint iced water
a few cubes of coarse brown
    bread

Chop the tomatoes until almost a purée. Stir in all the other ingredients. Keep very cold until it is time to serve the soup, then thin with the iced water, add the bread and serve with broken-up ice floating in the bowl. A couple of hard-boiled eggs, coarsely chopped, also make a good addition.

Grilled goats' cheese on bruschetta with roasted peppers

Toast pieces of foccacia bread (or French stick can be substituted). Cut some cloves of garlic in half and rub each piece of toast with a piece of it. This gives a good hint of garlic, without being overpowering. Brush each piece of toast with olive oil. Top the toasts with a thick round of goats' cheese, drizzle with more olive oil and grill until the top of the cheese bubbles. Serve with roasted peppers (see below) on a bed of rocket.

Roasted peppers

Cut peppers in half and remove the seeds and stems. Brush the peppers with oil and roast in a moderate oven until the skins have blackened. Peel the peppers by putting them in a plastic bag for ten minutes or so. The skins should then come off quite easily.

These can be prepared in advance, and stored in olive oil.

Garlic mushrooms

Serves 4

450 g / 1 lb mushrooms
175 g / 6 oz butter, at room
   temperature
2 cloves garlic, crushed
15 ml / 1 tbsp lemon juice

15–30 ml / 1–2 tbsp fresh
   chopped parsley
salt and freshly ground black
   pepper

Preheat oven to Gas Mark 7 / 220°C / 425°F. Prepare the mushrooms by simply wiping them with kitchen paper, then pull off the stalks – but don't discard them. In a small basin, combine the crushed garlic with the butter, and stir in the parsley and lemon juice. Season the mixture with salt and freshly ground black pepper.

Arrange the mushroom caps, skin side down, in a gratin dish or roasting tin, with the stalks arranged among them. Place a little of the garlic butter mixture into each cap, and spread whatever remains over the stalks as well.

Place the dish on the top shelf of the preheated oven, and cook for 10–15 minutes or until the butter is sizzling away and the mushrooms look slightly toasted. Serve straight from the oven with lashings of crusty bread to mop up the garlicky juices.

Aubergine dip

1 aubergine
1 red onion
$\frac{1}{2}$ green pepper
400 g/14 oz can chopped
  tomatoes
2 cloves garlic

1 dried long red chilli, seeds
  removed (optional)
generous spring of thyme
salt and pepper
olive oil

Dice the onion, aubergine and pepper. Sauté the onion with the finely chopped garlic. Add the aubergine, pepper, chopped chilli, thyme and salt and pepper. Stir. Add the tomatoes, cover and stew gently for about 40 minutes, stirring occasionally.

This is good either hot or cold, served as a dip, or as a filling for sandwiches. It is also good as a side vegetable dish, and the flavour improves after a day or two. The chilli will give it a kick, but isn't strictly necessary.

Aioli (garlic mayonnaise)

To prepare this classic garlic mayonnaise of Provence, make sure that all the ingredients are kept at room temperature for 1 hour beforehand.

Serves 6

10 garlic cloves
a little salt
1 ml/$\frac{1}{4}$ tsp finely ground black
  pepper

2 egg yolks
250 ml/8 fl oz olive oil
juice of 1 lemon
30 ml/2 tbsp lukewarm water

Peel the garlic cloves. Chop them coarsely and pound them in a mortar with the salt and pepper. Work in the egg yolks. Add the olive oil drop by drop, stirring all the time. When 60 ml/4 tbsp oil has been added, stir in the lemon juice and water. Continue adding more oil until the desired quantity of mayonnaise has been obtained. The finished product should be firmer than ordinary mayonnaise.

Tzatziki

The home-made version of this dip is much better than anything you can buy in the supermarket.

Peel, seed and grate a cucumber. Mix with some salt and leave it for half an hour. At the end of that time squeeze as much moisture as possible out of the cucumber. The drier it is the better. Crush 2 cloves of garlic and whisk them into 2 cups of Greek yogurt. Add 2 tablespoons finely chopped mint and 1 tablespoon finely chopped dill. Stir in the cucumber.

SALADS

Carrot, orange and tomato salad

This colourful salad is rich in vitamin C and beta carotene which is made into vitamin A by the body.

Serves 4

2 *large slicing tomatoes*
2 *large oranges*
2 *large carrots, peeled*
lettuce leaves

DRESSING
150 ml/$\frac{1}{4}$ pint olive oil
juice and grated rind of 1 orange
15 ml/1 tbsp wine vinegar
5 ml/1 tsp mild mustard
5 ml/1 tsp caster sugar
salt and freshly milled pepper

Skin, seed and cut the tomatoes into petals. Peel the oranges with a knife and cut into segments. Coarsely grate the carrots.

Make up the dressing by combining all the ingredients. Arrange the fruit and vegetables on lettuce leaves in individual bowls. Dress before serving or pass the dressing separately.

Winter salad with cheese

Serves 6

2 green peppers
2 red peppers
250 g/8 oz low-fat cheddar cheese

DRESSING
150 ml/¼ pint olive oil
30 ml/2 tbsp wine vinegar
1 clove garlic, crushed
5 ml/1 tsp mild mustard
salt and freshly milled pepper

Cut each pepper into fine strips. Cut the cheese into the same sized strips as the peppers. Chill in separate containers and mix together just before serving. Toss in the dressing just before serving.

Cheese, cucumber, tomato and orange salad

Serves 6

250 g/8 oz mature low-fat
 cheese, cut into cubes
2 large slicing tomatoes,
 skinned, seeded and cut into
 chunks

1 small cucumber, seeded and
 cut into chunks

DRESSING
150 ml/¼ pint olive oil
juice and finely grated rind of 1 orange
2.5 ml/½ tsp mild mustard
salt and freshly milled pepper
1 clove garlic, crushed (optional)
2.5 ml/½ tsp caster sugar

Put the dressing ingredients into a screw-topped jar and shake well. Mix the salad ingredients in a large bowl and chill. Dress the salad just before serving.

Chicory, red pepper and orange salad

Serves 4

2 heads chicory
1 red pepper
4 large sticks celery
1 large orange

DRESSING
60 ml / 4 tbsp olive oil
30 ml / 2 tbsp wine vinegar
5 ml / 1 tsp mild mustard
1 clove garlic, crushed
freshly ground black pepper

Cut each chicory head in half lengthways and then thinly slice it. Cut the pepper into strips. Chop the celery. Cut the rind and pith from the orange, cut the flesh into quarters lengthways and then thinly slice these. Mix together in a salad bowl.

Beat the remaining ingredients together and fold them into the salad.

Greek salad

Serves 4

2 large slicing tomatoes, cut into segments
half an onion, sliced finely
half a green pepper, sliced thinly
10 cm / 4 inch piece of cucumber, peeled and sliced

6–8 black or green olives
125 g / 4 oz feta cheese (rinsed briefly if too salty)
a pinch dried oregano
75 ml / 5 tbsp good quality olive oil
salt

Mix all the ingredients in a bowl and serve.

Green salad

Serves 4

1 small lettuce heart
1 small crisp lettuce
a quarter of a cucumber,
 sliced

4 spring onions
1 small bunch watercress
15 ml / 1 tbsp olive oil

DRESSING
15–30 ml / 1–2 tbsp lemon juice
large pinch mustard powder
5 ml/1 tsp clear honey
1 clove garlic, crushed
black pepper

Prepare the salad ingredients and chill. Just before serving, toss in the olive oil. Mix the dressing ingredients together and toss into the salad. Serve immediately.

Aubergine salad

Serves 6

750 g / 1½ lb aubergines
2 cloves garlic, sliced
juice of half a lemon, or more
    to taste

75 ml / 5 tbsp olive or good
    vegetable oil
salt and black pepper
black olives to garnish

Preheat the oven to Gas Mark 4 / 180°C / 350°F. Wash and dry the aubergines, prick them with a fork (otherwise they may explode in the oven) and cook them in the oven for one hour, turning them occasionally.

When the aubergines are cool enough to handle, halve them, scoop their flesh out into a sieve and press lightly to extract their bitter juices. Place their flesh, with the garlic and lemon juice, into a liquidizer and blend, adding the oil slowly at the same time, until quite smooth. Taste and adjust the seasoning, spread on a shallow platter and garnish with the olives.

MAIN DISHES

Stir-fried noodles

250 g/½ lb dried noodles
500 g/1 lb mixed vegetables
 cut into bite-sized pieces
 (baby sweetcorn, mangetout,
 peppers, mushrooms,
 beansprouts, pak choi, peas,
 carrot, broccoli – the choice
 is yours, limited only by
 what you like to eat)
½ an onion, finely diced

1–5 fresh green chillis,
 deseeded and sliced
a stick of lemongrass
3 cloves garlic
a piece of ginger, about the
 size of a plum
30 ml/2 tbsp light soy sauce
30 ml/2 tbsp fish sauce
5 ml/1 tsp sugar
oil

Cook the noodles, according to the instructions on the packet, while preparing and cooking the vegetables.

Pound the lemongrass, garlic and ginger in a mortar and pestle (or whizz up in the food processor). Heat a splash of oil in a wok. When it is very hot add the finely diced onion, and keep stirring. After a minute or so add the lemongrass, ginger and garlic, and keep stirring. (If it begins to stick add a bit of water.) Next put in all the vegetables and chilli and stir until heated through and cooked, but still crunchy. Add the drained noodles, which will be cooked by now, and splash in the soy sauce, fish sauce and sugar. Taste. You may want to add a bit more soy sauce and/or fish sauce.

This recipe has endless variations according to the sorts of vegetables you put in. The proportions of noodle to vegetable given are completely arbitrary – you may prefer more noodle and less vegetable. You can also use flat noodles for a change, and for an interesting variation take out the fish sauce and use oyster sauce instead. (If you are a strict vegetarian you won't want to use fish sauce or oyster sauce – just use some extra soy.)

Vegetable curry

1 large onion, diced
1 packet of frozen mixed
  vegetables
2 medium potatoes, diced
2 cloves garlic
a piece of ginger, about the
  size of a large grape
5 ml/1 tsp cumin

10 ml/2 tsp coriander
2.5 ml/$\frac{1}{2}$ tsp turmeric
2.5–10 ml/$\frac{1}{2}$–2 tsp chilli
  powder
5 ml/1 tsp salt
200 g/half a 14 oz can
  chopped tomatoes
vegetable oil

Fry the onion in the oil until transparent. Pound the garlic and ginger together in a mortar and pestle (or grate the ginger and crush the garlic). Add to the onion and cook for a minute or so. Add the cumin, coriander, turmeric, chilli powder and salt and stir for a minute (if it starts to stick add a little water). Add the frozen vegetables, potato and tomatoes and stir. Add enough water to not quite cover the vegetables and simmer for 20–30 minutes, until the vegetables are cooked.

Carrot and courgette stew

Serves 4

250 g/½ lb carrots, sliced
  5 mm/¼ inch thick
500 g/1 lb small courgettes,
  sliced 5 mm/¼ inch thick
100 g/4 oz butter

4 tomatoes (350 g/12 oz
  approx) peeled and chopped
salt, sugar and pepper
extra knob of butter
parsley, chopped

Blanch the carrots in boiling salted water for 3 minutes. Add the courgettes, and boil for a further 3–5 minutes until the vegetables are half cooked. Drain well.

Melt the butter in a large heavy frying pan. Add the carrots and courgettes. Cook gently, stirring often, for 10 minutes. Add the tomatoes and continue cooking.

When the tomatoes are reduced to a thick buttery sauce and the vegetables are done, correct the seasoning, and stir in the extra butter. Sprinkle with parsley and serve.

Curried carrots

Serves 4

750 g / 1½ lbs carrots, sliced
  diagonally
50 g / 2 oz onion, chopped
1 clove garlic, chopped
50 g / 2 oz butter
30 ml / 2 rounded tbsp flour

15 ml / 1 tbsp curry powder
1 eating apple, cored and
  diced
200 g / 8 oz low-fat fromage
  frais
salt and pepper

Cook the carrots in an inch of boiling, salted water. Drain, and keep the cooking water. Soften the onion and garlic in the butter. Stir in the flour and curry powder. Moisten with carrot water. Add the apple and fromage frais. Simmer for 15 minutes at least. Check the seasoning and the consistency of the sauce, then serve in a ring of boiled, buttered rice.

Vegetable mixed grill

Serves 4

8 *medium open mushrooms*	1 *medium aubergine (350 g /*
4 *tomatoes*	*12 oz approx)*
4 *small courgettes*	

MARINADE
125 ml / 4 fl oz olive oil
juice of a lemon
30 ml / 2 tbsp tomato purée
10 ml / 2 tsp paprika
a pinch chilli powder
30 ml / 2 tbsp chopped fresh thyme
or 10 ml / 2 tsp dried thyme

Trim the stalks of the mushrooms, leaving only about 5 mm / $\frac{1}{4}$ inch. Halve the tomatoes crossways and cut each courgette in half lengthways. Cut the aubergine into 8 slices of equal thickness.

Mix the ingredients for the marinade together. Turn the mushrooms, courgettes and aubergines in the marinade and leave them for 30 minutes. Just before cooking, brush the marinade over the tomatoes.

Heat the grill to high. Grill the courgettes for 2 minutes on each side, the aubergines for about $1\frac{1}{2}$ minutes on each side, the mushrooms for $1\frac{1}{2}$ minutes each side, and the tomatoes, cut side up only, for 2 minutes. Arrange the cooked vegetables attractively on a serving plate.

Spanish tortilla

This is a basic Spanish omelette. It is best made in a frying pan with curved or sloping sides.

2 *medium potatoes*	*salt and pepper*
5 *eggs*	*vegetable oil*
$\frac{1}{2}$ *cup milk*	

Cut the potato into a small dice and fry the oil. Beat the eggs with the milk, add the cooked potato and some salt and pepper. Heat some oil in the frying pan and add the egg mixture. Cook on a medium heat. When the bottom of the omelette is set, turn it over and cook the other side. Turning the omelette can be awkward. The Spanish have a trick which involves upending the frying pan onto a large plate, then sliding the omelette back in. You can also put the pan under a grill to cook the top half.

This is another dish with endless variations. Try adding some cheese and ham, or steamed asparagus or broccoli. Spinach or leeks are also good.

PASTA AND RICE

Basic risotto

500 g/1 lb arborio rice
1.5 litres/3 pints vegetable
  stock
a small onion, finely diced
a pinch of saffron, soaked for
  10 minutes in a little water

125 g/4 oz unsalted butter
90 g/3 oz grated Parmesan
  cheese

Heat the stock in a saucepan, and keep warm over a low heat. Sauté
the onion slowly in half the butter until it is translucent. Add the rice
and stir until it is coated with the butter. Add the saffron and the
water in which it is soaking. Add a ladle of warm vegetable stock
and stir until it is all absorbed. Gradually add the rest of the stock,
stirring occasionally until the rice is cooked. This should take about
20 minutes. When the rice is cooked add the rest of the butter and
the Parmesan cheese.

Risotto is another of those useful dishes which can be varied
endlessly. Vegetables which go well with risotto include mushrooms, leeks, butternut squash, peppers or spinach. Tarragon, thyme
or parsley also enhance the flavour. Left-over risotto can be made
into rice patties. Mix the cold risotto with a beaten egg or two, form
into patties and shallow fry. Alternatively shape the rice mixture into
balls around small cubes of mozzarella cheese, deep fry and serve
with a fresh green salad.

Pasta with tomato and egg sauce

Serves 4

2 large onions, sliced
15 ml / 1 tbsp olive oil
two 400 g / 14 oz cans chopped
  tomatoes
300 g / 10 oz wholemeal or
  spinach (green) pasta shapes

15 ml / 1 tbsp chopped fresh
  basil
3 eggs, beaten lightly
fresh Parmesan cheese, grated
salt and pepper

Cook the onions very slowly in the olive oil. They should become soft but not coloured and this should take 15–20 minutes. Add the tomatoes, salt and pepper, stir well and bring the mixture up to the boil. Let it simmer for 10 minutes.

Meanwhile, cook the pasta in rapidly boiling water to which a teaspoon of oil and a little salt has been added. When the pasta is cooked, drain it well and refresh with hot water.

Take the tomato sauce off the heat, check the seasoning, add the basil and then gradually pour in the lightly beaten eggs. The sauce should become rich and creamy.

Mix a little of the sauce with the pasta, pile it into a serving dish and pour the remaining sauce over it. Serve sprinkled with a little freshly grated Parmesan cheese.

Wholemeal tagliatelle with peppers

Peppers are a good source of vitamin A.

Serves 4

1 red pepper	*60 ml/4 tbsp grated Parmesan*
1 yellow pepper	*cheese*
2 cloves garlic, sliced	*a small bunch of coriander,*
90 ml/6 tbsp olive oil	*chopped finely*
450 g/1 lb wholemeal	*salt and freshly ground black*
tagliatelle	*pepper*

Cut the peppers into quarters and grill them skin-side up until the skins blister and can be easily peeled off. Cut into strips.

Cook the garlic gently in 30 ml/2 tbsp of the oil until soft, then stir in the peppers and cook for a minute or two. Season generously with salt and pepper, and add the rest of the oil.

Boil the tagliatelle, drain and then toss in the pepper mixture. Stir in the grated cheese and coriander, adjust the seasoning and serve at once.

Pasta in ginger and tomato sauce

Serves 4

10 ml / 2 tsp olive oil
1 onion, finely chopped
4 celery sticks, trimmed and
  finely chopped
30 ml / 2 tbsp finely chopped
  fresh root ginger
two 400 g / 14 oz cans peeled
  tomatoes

10 ml / 2 tsp chopped
  marjoram
45 ml / 3 tbsp tomato purée
375 g / 12 oz wholemeal
  macaroni
5 ml / 1 tsp lemon juice
salt and pepper
grated Parmesan cheese
chopped fresh parsley

For the sauce, heat the oil in a medium-sized saucepan and gently fry the onion and celery for 5 minutes until soft. Add the ginger and cook gently for a further 2 minutes to allow the flavours to blend.

Add the tomatoes, marjoram and tomato purée. Bring to the boil. Reduce the heat and simmer for 15 minutes until the tomatoes are cooked.

Meanwhile, cook the macaroni by simmering in $2\frac{1}{2}$ litres / 4 pints water with a little lemon juice for 10 minutes. When it is cooked, drain well, mix with the sauce, season and serve garnished with Parmesan and chopped parsley.

Garlic and broccoli spaghetti

Serves 4–5

500 g / 1 lb sprouting broccoli
300 g / 10 oz spaghetti
105 ml / 7 tbsp virgin olive oil
2–3 cloves garlic, finely
  chopped

sea salt and black pepper
freshly grated Parmesan cheese
  (optional)

Wash the broccoli and cut into 1 cm / $\frac{1}{2}$ inch pieces, discarding any hard, thick stalks. Put a little salted water in a saucepan and bring it to the boil. Add the broccoli, cover the pan and boil for only 2 minutes. Drain.

Heat a large pan of salted water and when boiling add the spaghetti.

Meanwhile, heat the olive oil in a large frying pan, add the garlic and cook over a low heat for a minute or two until just browned. Add the broccoli and stir it around over the heat for a minute. Sprinkle with sea salt and plenty of black pepper and turn off the heat.

The spaghetti should be ready in 7–10 minutes, perhaps less if it is fresh; it should be cooked through but still with a slight bite to it. Drain and rinse through with running hot water, then put it into a warmed serving bowl. Mix in the broccoli and garlic and serve immediately. Have the sea salt and black pepper grinders on the table to season if needed, and a bowl of freshly grated Parmesan cheese to sprinkle over if you like.

A useful tomato sauce

two 400 g/14 oz cans chopped   2 cloves garlic, crushed
   tomatoes   olive oil
1 medium onion, diced

Sauté the onion and garlic in a splash of olive oil until it is soft and translucent. Add the tomatoes, some salt and pepper, and simmer for 10 minutes.

This can be served on pasta as it is, but it can also be varied. Try adding some basil and oregano, or capers and chopped olives, or some sliced fresh chillis, or mushrooms. If you are not vegetarian a tin of tuna thrown in is popular with children.

SIDE DISHES

Ratatouille

Serves 4

15 ml / 1 tbsp olive oil
1 onion, chopped
2 cloves garlic, crushed
1 medium aubergine, diced
4 courgettes, sliced
2 red peppers, deseeded and
* diced*

400 g / 14 oz can tomatoes
1 bay leaf
sprig of fresh thyme
salt and pepper

Heat the oil in a pan and gently fry the onion for a few minutes. Add the garlic, aubergine, courgettes and peppers. Cook for 10 minutes, stirring occasionally.

Add the tomatoes and herbs and cook gently for 40 minutes until the vegetables are fairly soft. Season and serve.

Aubergine and mushroom rice

Serves 4

250 g / 8 oz brown long-grain
* rice*
10 ml / 2 tsp olive oil
1 large onion
1 large clove garlic, chopped
375 g / 12 oz aubergine, diced
125 g / 4 oz mushrooms,
* quartered*

10 ml / 2 tsp chopped fresh
* marjoram*
10 ml / 2 tsp chopped fresh
* thyme*
5 ml / 1 tsp paprika
25 g / 1 oz wholemeal flour
300 ml / $\frac{1}{2}$ pint skimmed milk
15 ml / 1 tbsp soy sauce

Place the rice in 600 ml / 1 pint boiling water. Bring back to the boil, cover and simmer for 25 minutes. Drain and transfer the rice to a large casserole or ovenproof dish.

Heat the oil and gently fry the onion and garlic for 5 minutes. Add the aubergine and mushrooms and cook for a further 10 minutes.

Add the marjoram, thyme, paprika and flour and cook for 2–3 minutes. Add the milk and simmer for 5 minutes. Add the soy sauce and check the seasoning.

Put the aubergine mixture on top of the rice. Cover and bake in a preheated oven at Gas Mark 4 / 180°C / 350°F for 30 minutes. Serve hot.

Carrots with garlic and ginger

Serves 3–4

15 ml / 1 tbsp cumin seeds
450 g / 1 lb young carrots,
  sliced
1 large clove garlic, crushed

2.5 cm / 1 inch piece of root
  ginger, peeled and grated
30 ml / 2 tbsp soy sauce

Preheat the oven to Gas Mark 5 / 190°C / 375°F. Put the cumin seeds on a baking tray and cook for 5 minutes until lightly toasted, shaking them around from time to time. Put to one side.

Steam the carrots in a colander or steamer over simmering water until they are cooked but still crunchy. Mix the garlic and ginger into the soy sauce and toss the carrots in it, mixing well. Sprinkle with the cumin seeds just before serving.

Potatoes cooked with rosemary and garlic

Splash some olive oil into the bottom of a roasting tin and put into a very hot oven until it is hot. Take about 750 g / 1½ lb of new potatoes and cut into large dice (each piece of potato should be roughly the size of a plum). Toss the potatoes into the hot oil, add a head of garlic cloves, unpeeled, throw on a generous amount of rosemary, freshly ground black pepper and some sea salt. Bake in the hot oven until the outside is browned and crunchy. You'll probably need to turn them once during cooking. This is particularly popular with children.

Aubergine purée

2 medium aubergines
olive oil, cumin, salt and pepper to taste

Peel the aubergines and bake them in a moderate oven, seasoned
with the other ingredients, until soft. Purée in a blender, adding extra
oil and seasoning to achieve a smooth consistency.

An alternative to chips

Take some parsnip, beetroot or butternut squash, cut into thin slices
and deep fry. Sprinkle with sea salt and eat either hot or cold.

Useful Addresses

The Anaphylaxis Campaign
PO Box 149
Fleet
Hants GU13 0FA
Tel. 01252 542029
Fax 01252 377140
Website www.anaphylaxis.org.uk

The British Allergy Foundation
Deepdene House
30 Bellegrove Road
Welling
Kent DA16 3PY
Tel. 020 8303 8525
Helpline 020 8303 8792
Fax 020 8303 8583
Email baf@nascr.net
Website
www.allergyfoundation.com

British Lung Foundation
78 Hatton Garden
London EC1N 8LD
Tel. 020 7831 5831
Fax 020 7831 5832
Email blf_user@gpiag-asthma.org
Website www.lunguk.org

Medic Alert Foundation
1 Bridge Wharf
156 Caledonian Road
London N1 9UU
Tel. 020 7833 3034
Linkline 0800 581420
Fax 020 7713 5653
Email info@medicalert.co.uk
Website www.medicalert.co.uk

National Asthma Campaign
Providence House
Providence Place
London N1 0NT
Tel. 020 7226 2260
Helpline 0845 7010203
Fax 020 7704 0740
Website www.asthma.org.uk

National Eczema Society
163 Eversholt Street
London NW1 1BU
Tel. 020 7388 4097
Helpline 0870 241 3604
Fax 020 7388 5882
Website www.eczema.org

Further Reading

Clough, Dr Joanne, *Allergies at your Fingertips* (Class Publishing, 1997).

Davies, Dr Stephen, and Stewart, Dr Alan, *Nutritional Medicine* (Pan Books, 1987).

Williams, Dr Deryk, Williams, Anna, and Croker, Laura, *Life-threatening Allergic Reactions* (Piatkus Books, 1997).

Index

adrenaline (epinephrine):
administering 14–15, 24,
34–5
Aioli (garlic mayonnaise) 59
airline travel 27
allergic reaction *see*
anaphylaxis
allergies: antibodies 8–9;
becoming sensitized 5;
immune system 7; lifelong
condition 32; self-defence
24–5; types of reaction 8–9
allergy testing 9–10; blood
(RAST and CAP-RAST)
10–11; 'challenge' in
hospital 31; skin-prick 10,
32–3
almonds 29
alternative chips 80
anaphylaxis 3; confusion with
heart attack 36; emergency
action 14–16; emergency
reaction 15–16; symptoms
13–14; whole body response
33–4
*Anaphylaxis: Guidance for
Carers of Pre-School
Children* (Anaphylaxis
Campaign) 31
*Anaphylaxis and Schools: How
We Can Make It Work*
(Anaphylaxis Campaign)
31–2
Anaphylaxis Campaign 3–4;

*Anaphylaxis: Guidance for
Carers of Pre-School
Children* 31; *Anaphylaxis
and Schools: How We Can
Make It Work* 31–2
asthma 33, 37–41; control
38–9; nuts worsen symptoms
35
'atopic' people 5, 30
aubergines: dip 58; and
mushroom rice 78–9; puréed
80; salad 65

Baillie, Ross 4
brazil nuts 29
British Allergy Foundation 33
Brostoff, Jonathan: *The
Complete Guide to Food
Allergy and Intolerance*
(with Gamlin) 47

carrots: and courgette stew 68;
curried 69; with garlic and
ginger 79; orange and
tomato salad 61
cheese, cucumber, tomato and
orange salad 62
chicory, red pepper and orange
salad 63
Christmas food 55
coconut 21–2
complementary medicine 36
*The Complete Guide to Food
Allergy and Intolerance*
(Brostoff and Gamlin) 47

convenience foods: 'may contain' labels 30; reading labels 19–22
cosmetics 28–9
cot death 36

eczema 35–6, 41–4; relation to asthma 40; treatments 44; types 43–4
eggs 3
emotions: bottled up 11–12; coping with the risks 25–6; embarrassment 26
exercise 11

fats 50
fish 48, 49
food intolerances 46–7
fruit and vegetables: Mediterranean diet 47–8; nutritional need 49, 51–2

Gamlin, Linda: *The Complete Guide to Food Allergy and Intolerance* (with Brostoff) 47
garlic 51
Garlic: and broccoli spaghetti 76; mushrooms 58; soup 56
Gazpacho 57
Greek salad 63
Green salad 63
Grilled goats' cheese on bruschetta 57

hay fever 44–5
hazelnuts 29
holidays 33

immune system 7; looking after 11–12

immunoglobulin E (IgE) 8–9
insect stings 3

laughter 12
legumes: overlap with peanut allergies 33

Medic Alert 27, 33
milk 3

nut allergies: overlap 35
nutmeg 22
nutrition: ingredients of 49–52; meat 51; the Mediterranean diet 47–8; restricting calories 50; for vegetarians 48–9; well-balanced diet 11
nuts: key points in avoiding 46; Latin names 29; nutritional value 3; pre-packaged foods 19–22

oils 20–1

Pasta: in ginger and tomato sauce 75; with tomato and egg sauce 73
peanuts 4; Latin ingredient name 29; other legumes 33; pre-packaged food 19–21; widespread use 4–5
Peppers, roasted 57
poppy seeds 4
Potatoes cooked with rosemary and garlic 79
pregnancy and breastfeeding 5, 30–1
Pumpkin soup with cumin and ginger 56

Ratatouille 78

Reading, David 25–6
Reading, Sarah 3, 25
restaurant food 22–4
Risotto, basic 72
rubber (latex) 3

schools and pre-schools 31–2
Seed Crushers and Oil
    Processors Association
    (SCOPA) 21
seeds: overlaps with nuts
    allergies 4
sesame seeds 3, 4, 33; Latin
    name 29; pre-packaged
    foods 22
shellfish 3
sleep 11
soya 3
soya bean foods 50
Spanish tortilla 71
spices: seed allergies 4
Stir-fried noodles 66
stress 11
sugar 11, 51

*Supporting pupils with medical
    needs in school* (DfEE/DoH)
    32

Thrasher, Laura 4
Tomato sauce 77
Tzatziki 60

urticaria 45

Vegetable: curry 67; mixed
    grill 70
vegetables: *see* fruit and
    vegetables
vegetarians: nutrition 48–9

walnuts 29
water, drinking 49–50
Wholemeal tagliatelle with
    peppers 74
Winter salad with cheese 62

yoghurt 11